Clinical Ocular Phys

An introductory text

To my wife, Mandy

Clinical Ocular Physiology
An introductory text

by

N. H. Victor Chong MB ChB(Glasgow), DO(Ireland),
FRCSEd, FRCOphth
Institute of Ophthalmology, London

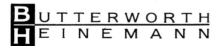

Butterworth-Heinemann
Linacre House, Jordan Hill, Oxford OX2 8DP
A division of Reed Educational and Professional Publishing Ltd

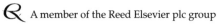 A member of the Reed Elsevier plc group

OXFORD   BOSTON   JOHANNESBURG
MELBOURNE   NEW DELHI   SINGAPORE

First published 1996

British Library Cataloguing in Publication Data
Chong, Victor
    Clinical ocular physiology: an introductory text
    1 Eye – Physiology   2 Ophthalmology
    I. Title
    612.8′4

ISBN 0 7506 2718 2

Library of Congress Cataloguing in Publication Data
Chong, N. H. Victor.
    Clinical ocular physiology: an introductory text/by N.H. Victor Chong
    p. cm.
    Includes index.
    ISBN 0 7506 2718 2
    1. Eye – Physiology.   I. Title
    [DNLM: 1. Eye – physiology.   2. Vision – physiology.   WW 103 C548c]
    QP475.C48
    612.8′4–dc20

                                                                    96–20041
                                                                    CIP

Origination by David Gregson Associates, Beccles, Suffolk
Printed and bound in Great Britain by Biddles Ltd, Guildford and King's Lynn

Contents

Foreword

There is increasing common ground between visual scentists and those working in clinical ophthalmology. With the recent advances in the appreciation of disease mechanisms in Ophthalmology, a good understanding of the physiology of the eye and the visual system is becoming progressively more important to clinicians. This is exemplified by the impact of molecular genetics upon our understanding of inherited retinal dystrophies and their management. It was particularly fortunate that there was good understanding of phototransduction such that it was possible to form concepts as to the potential influence of mutations on protein structure and function within the photoreceptor cell. Tests of retinal function exist allowing the characterization of visual loss consequent upon the mutations.

All of us have been intimidated by voluminous texts of ophthalmic physiology in our early careers in clinical ophthalmology. It is difficult to know where to start, and to determine what is very important and what is less so. This text is intended to provide a framework which is brief and easy to understand, and important attributes have been highlighted. It is hoped that as an introductory text, it will allow an overview that will be useful to those starting out in their career. It is by no means comprehensive and is not intended to be so. Some sections are simplified to highlight important principles. It is believed that having read this book, longer texts will be easier to tackle given a skeleton on which to build.

Professor Alan C Bird MD FRCS FRCOphth
Institute of Ophthalmology, Moorfields Eye Hospital, London

Preface

Many people struggle to find an appropriate introductory text-book in ocular physiology: clinical books do not have sufficient basic ocular physiology, whilst standard ocular physiology books are written by research scientists for physiologists. It is my aim to fill the gap between these two extremes.

Ocular physiology is an important, interesting subject and the basic background knowledge allows us to understand the pathophysiology of disease and to rationalize its management. In clinical practice, some physiological facts might not be important but would be of interest: for instance, fluorescein is frequently used by ophthalmologists and optometrists in looking for corneal epithelial defects; but what does it stain? Certainly not dead cells, or corneal epithelial cells! The answer is in this book.

There are four main sections: section A presents basic ocular physiology based on anatomical division, section B discusses physiological topics concerning visual function. Section C examines important associated disciplines and section D discusses basic principles of ophthalmic investigations and lasers.

This book was written particularly for ophthalmic trainees and student optometrists. It would be of interest to ophthalmologists, optometrists, orthoptists, ophthalmic nurses, physiology students and senior medical students.

I am extremely grateful to my former colleagues Chris Gordon, Prue Dobinson and Louise Field in optometry, orthoptics and ophthalmic nursing respectively for their valuable criticism and suggestions. Special thanks to Louise for her painstaking effort in checking the whole manuscript and to my wife, Mandy, for her whole-hearted support. Last but not least, I am indebted to Professor Alan Bird for his foreword.

Section A
Ocular physiology

Chapter 1

Eyelids

The eyelids form one of the most important elements in the ocular protective system. Starting from the eyelashes, they provide a mechanical screen for dust and dirt. Reflex blinking protects the eyes by lid closure from various potentially harmful stimuli such as approaching objects and bright light. Spontaneous blinking spreads the precorneal tear film to improve lubrication of the ocular surfaces. Finally, the oily layer and part of the aqueous layer of the precorneal tear film are secreted by the lids.

Protective mechanisms

- Physical screening by the eyelashes.
- Blinking movement of the eyelids.
- Secretions of the glands in the eyelids.

Normal eyelid movement

Lid opening

Upper lid elevators

Elevation of the upper lid is mainly controlled by the levator muscle. Muller's and frontalis muscles play their own role and become important when the levator is defective. The attachments and nerve supply of these muscles are summarized in Table 1.1.

Table 1.1 The upper lid elevators

Muscle	Attachments	Nerve supply
Levator palpebrae superioris	Lesser wing of the sphenoid to the tarsal plate	Oculomotor nerve (CNIII)
Muller's muscles	Aponeurosis of the levator to the upper border of the tarsal plate	Sympathetic
Frontalis	Scalp to the upper part of the orbicularis oculi	Facial nerve (CNVII)

Lower lid retractors

A fibrous tissue sheet (as compared with the aponeurosis of the levator) extends from the sheath of the inferior rectus muscle to the lower border of the tarsal plate. It is accompanied by the inferior tarsal muscle (as compared with the Muller's muscle).

Lid closure

Orbicularis oculi controls lid closure and is supplied by the facial nerve (CNVII) It is divided into three main parts as summarized in Table 1.2.

Table 1.2 Orbicularis muscle

Part	Position	Function
Orbital	Surrounds the orbital rims	Forced lid closure
Preseptal	In front of the orbital septum	Pull lacrimal fascia laterally and create a relative vacuum in lacrimal sac—improve tear drainage
Pretarsal	In front of the tarsal plate	Close lid and pull lacrimal puncta medially

Involutional changes of the lids in the elderly

- The preseptal muscle can move upwards over the pretarsal muscle, leading to the inward turning of the lower lid (entropion).
- Lower lid retractor laxity allows the lower border of the tarsal plate to rotate outward combining with an atrophic tarsal plate. The lid loses its stiffness and can turn inward (entropion) or outward (ectropion).
- Horizontal lid laxity is caused by combined atrophic changes in the orbicularis, canthal tendons and tarsal plate. This is aggravated by relative enophthalmos secondary to atrophic orbital fat. The lid can turn inward or outward.

Clinical points

Correction of involutional entropion and ectropion is the most commonly performed eyelid surgery. The type of procedure required would depend on the main involutional changes of the patient. It is vital to correct the abnormalities present.

In general, entropion is corrected by everting sutures which turn the lid to the correct position, combined with a horizontal lid split stopping the preseptal muscle moving upwards (Wies procedure). This can be combined with horizontal lid shortening (Quickert procedure) in reducing lid and tarsal plate laxity. Ectropion can usually be corrected by horizontal lid shortening alone by wedge resection.

Blinking

There are two main types of blinking: reflex blinking is induced by certain stimuli, and protects the eye from the threatening stimulus, whilst spontaneous blinking is an involuntary lid movement.

Reflex blinking

This is a voluntary reflex secondary to various stimuli. Different stimuli induce a different neurological pathway; these are summarized in Table 1.3.

Table 1.3 The blinking reflexes. CN II = optic nerve, CNV = trigeminal nerve, CNVII = facial nerve, CNVIII = auditory nerve.

Blinking reflex	Examples	Afferent	Efferent	Central connection
Tactile	Corneal touch	CNV	CNVII	Cortical
Dazzle	Bright light	CNII	CNVII	Subcortical
Menace	Sudden presence of near object	CNII	CNVII	Cortical
Auditory	Loud noise	CNVIII	CNVII	Subcortical
Orbicularis	Stretching of panorbital structure	CNV	CNVII	Cortical

Clinical points

Contact lens wearers develop reduced or even absent tactile corneal reflexes. This allows for better contact lens tolerance.

Patients with essential blepharospasm have uncontrollable frequent blinking. It is disabling and unsightly for the patient. In the past, it was difficult to treat. Some surgeons had considered local facial nerve resection, although this may lead to permanent facial palsy. Another option is orbicularis resection.

The condition is now successfully treated by multiple subcutaneous injections of Botulinum toxin around the eye. This blocks the nerve action for about 3–6 months. In a lower dosage, a compromise can be achieved by the reduction of blepharospasm without affecting voluntary eyelid movements.

Spontaneous blinking

- Normal blinking during waking hours.
- Blink rate is specific to each individual.
- Average rate: 15 times per minute.
- Duration: 0.3–0.4 s.
- Present in the blind — hence no retinal stimulation is required.
- No discontinuity of visual sensation during blinking.
- The upper lid begins to close with no lower lid movement.
- It is followed by a zipper-like movement from the lateral canthus towards the medical canthus.
- This helps the displacement of the tear film to the lacrimal puncta which are located on the medial side of the lids.

Secretions of the eyelids

The eyelids contain various glands (see Figure 1.1) which secrete the different layers of the precorneal tear film. The details are summarized in Table 1.4. A detailed description of the precorneal tear film can be found in Chapter 2.

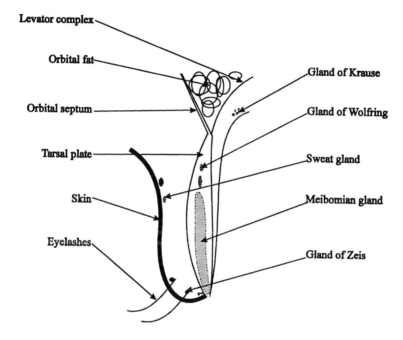

Figure 1.1 Cross-section of the upper eyelids showing the positions of various glands

Table 1.4 Secretion of the eyelids

Glands	Tear film layer	Location of glands
Meibomian glands	Oily layer	Tarsal plate
Glands of Zeis	Oily layer	Eyelashes
Glands of Wolfring	Aqueous layer	Tarsal plate
Glands of Krause	Aqueous layer	Fornix

Chapter 2

Lacrimal apparatus and tear film

Outline

The precorneal tear film plays a major role in the optical function of the eye. In order to achieve a balance of adequate lubrication without spillage, effective secretory and excretory mechanisms are required.

Lacrimal glands, accessory lacrimal glands, Meibomian glands and goblet cells on the conjunctiva secrete the different components of the tear film. About 10–25% of tear fluid is lost through evaporation; the remaining fluid drains through the lacrimal puncta on the medial side of the lids, from where it drains into the nose through the lacrimal canaliculi, lacrimal sac and nasolacrimal duct.

The surface area of the conjunctiva and cornea is about 16 cm^2. The volume of the tear film is about 7–9 µl normally but the eye can manage up to 30 µl without overflow. The turnover rate is 0.1–0.15 µl per minute. The overall thickness of the tear film is about 4–9 µm and thickest after blinking.

Function of the tear film

The function of the tear film is to:

- Maintain an optically uniform corneal surface.
- Flush cellular debris and foreign material from the cornea and conjunctival sac.
- Lubricate the corneal and conjunctival surfaces.
- Provide nutrients to the cornea.
- Provide antibacterial protection.

Structure of the tear film

- Anterior lipid layer.
- Middle aqueous layer.
- Mucoid layer.

The function and origin of the different layers in the precorneal tear film are summarized in Table 2.1.

Table 2.1 The precorneal tear film

	Lipid	*Aqueous*	*Mucoid*
Location	Anterior	Middle	Epithelial
Thickness	0.1 µm	6.5–7.5 µm	0.02–0.05 µm
Secreted by	Meibomian glands, glands of Zeis	Lacrimal glands, accessory glands of Krause and Wolfring	Goblet cells in conjunctiva
Function	Reduces evaporation, prevent overflow from lid margins	Contains nutrients and uptakes oxygen for cornea	Allows the tear film to spread evenly on a hydrophobic surface

Clinical points

- The pH is about 7.4 but becomes more acidic in inflammation and lid closure.
- The oxygen tension is about 140–160 mmHg. That can be reduced to 20 mmHg with a tightly fitting contact lens. Corneal oedema may occur if the oxygen tension is under 74 mmHg.

- Sjogren's syndrome with reduced production in the aqueous component of tears can cause hypertonicity, leading to corneal dehydration. Hypotonic eyedrops alone can provide relief by reducing the hypertonicity; however, tear-replacement eye drops can also stabilize the tear film.
- The corneal epithelial surface has fine microvilli, which increase the surface area and provide a greater area for attachment of the tear film. Corneal scars or other corneal abnormalities may result in patches of localized corneal drying.

Composition of tears

It is an obsession to many MCQ examiners to ask about the relative difference between the tears and the plasma. The clinical importance is very small if any. Instead of giving a list of figures which can be found in most standard textbooks, Table 2.2 gives an approximate percentage of the relative amount between the two. For instance, there is about 20 mmol/l of potassium in tears compared with 5 mmol/l in plasma; Table 2.2 shows this difference as 400%. In the case of sodium, there is 140 mmol/l in both tears and plasma, and a figure of 100% is shown.

Table 2.2 Composition of tears

Properties or components	Tears/plasma (%)	Reason for difference (if known)
pH	100	
Refractive index	100	
Bicarbonate	110	Indicates active secretion by lacrimal gland
Chloride	125	Indicates active secretion by lacrimal gland
Potassium	400	Indicates active secretion by lacrimal gland
Sodium	100	
Total protein	10	
Total nitrogen	10	Less metabolic wastes
Glucose	4	Less metabolic needs

Immunoglobulins in tears

- Overall Ig level is less in tears.
- The IgG/IgA ratios differ between tears and plasma; it is about 7:1 in plasma but almost 1:1 in tears.
- IgA has an additional 'secretory piece' molecule in tears.
- It is believed that secretory IgA is locally produced in the lacrimal gland rather than being a transudate from the serum.

Enzymes in tears

- The concentration of lysozyme in tears is higher than in any other body fluids.
- Lysozyme is a long-chain, high-molecular weight proteolytic enzyme produced by lysosome, an intracellular structure.
- It dissolves bacterial walls by enzymatic digestion.
- Lysozyme level is reduced in Sjogren's (dry eye) syndrome and this fact has been used as a diagnostic test.
- Beta-lysin is another bactericidal protein found in tears.
- It acts in the cellular membrane.

Secretion of tears

Tear secretion can be classified as basal secretion or reflex secretion, which can be central or peripheral. The details are summarized in Table 2.3.

Table 2.3 **Secretion of tears**

	Basal secretion	*Reflex section of peripheral origin*	*Reflex secretion of central origin*
Stimulus	None required	Stimulation of cornea, conjunctiva	Light, psychogenic
Afferent pathway	None	Trigeminal nerve	Cortical, brain stem
Control system	Sympathetic	Parasympathetic	Parasympathetic
Efferent pathway	Superior cervical ganglion	Sphenopalatine ganglion	Sphenopalatine ganglion
Main source of secretion	Accessory lacrimal glands and eyelids glands	Lacrimal gland	Lacrimal gland

Elimination of tears

- Evaporation — about 10–25% of tears are lost in this way.
- Blinking increases the pressure within the conjunctival sac at the same time at which a relative vacuum is formed in the lacrimal sac.
- It is disputable which of these two factors is more important in tears elimination from the conjunctival sac.

- Lacrimal canaliculi — capillary attraction plays a role in pulling tears into the sac.
- Nasolacrimal duct — once in the sac, gravity takes the tears down to the nose and reflux is prevented by an internal valve system.

Clinical points

Dry eyes and watery eyes are one of the most common presenting complaints to an eye department. Management can be very difficult unless a diagnosis is made. In some situations, the symptoms may not improve. Nevertheless it is important to give the patient a full explanation, reassurance and treatment option for their condition.

Clinical evaluation for dry eyes and watery eyes

Careful history taking with slit-lamp examination is most important. For instance, intermittent watery eyes are occasionally associated with naso-lacrimal duct blockage.

Slit-lamp examination

It is crucial to look for lid margin diseases as well as local allergic responses. A small subtarsal foreign body is an uncommon cause of persistent watery eye, yet it would be an unforgiveable mistake to miss it. With practice, examining the lid margin tear strip would give the examiner a good idea of how dry the eye is.

Tear film break-up time (BUT)

Deficiencies of the mucous layer of the tear film reduce the stability of the tear film. Hence, dry spots on the corneal surface appear quickly after blinking. The normal BUT is about 15–35 seconds. It is considered to be abnormal if it is less than 10 s. Traditionally, it is tested by putting fluorescein into the conjunctival sac. The first appearance of dry spots after a blink is timed and observed using the cobalt blue illumination in the slit-lamp. With modern slit-lamps and higher magnification, fluorescein is not required in many cases.

Schirmer test

Schirmer devised this test in 1903. A filter paper strip is folded and hung over the lower eyelids. The moistening of the exposed paper strip over a 5-minute period forms a measure of the rate of tear secretion. If the test is performed after a topical anaesthetic, only the basic secretion is measured. Values of less than 5 mm are commonly considered to be abnormal. The reflex secretion (Schirmer II test) can be measured by repeating the process while stimulating the nasal mucosa with chemical or mechanical irritants.

With practice, it is not difficult to assess the stability of the tear film by examining the lid margin tear strip and the tear film break-up time during slit-lamp examination. Schirmer tests are seldomly required in clinical practice.

Probing and syringing (sac wash-out)

After dilating the punctum and canaliculus, a lacrimal cannula is passed into the lacrimal sac. The cannula can be stopped by a common canalicular membrane (rare) which would feel elastic and it is described as 'soft stop'. More commonly, the cannula is stopped by the bone, the 'hard stop'. Once the cannula is in the sac, saline is injected slowly down the naso-lacrimal duct. The patient should be able to feel the saline on the back of the throat if the duct is patent. In total obstruction, all the saline would reflux back into the eye through the other canaliculus. If a mucocele is present, the regurgitated fluid might be purulent. The presence of a mucocele is often an indication for surgery and it carries a better result.

Jones dye test

A drop of 2% fluorescein is instilled into the conjunctival sac. A small cotton bud moistened with adrenaline and cocaine is inserted into the nose to recover the dye. In a normal system, it should be recovered within 5 minutes (Jones I test). A positive test indicates a normal system; however, over 20% of normal patients give a negative test.

If the Jones I test is negative, the Jones II test is performed. Residual fluorescein is flushed from the conjunctival sac after 5 minutes and clear saline solution is instilled into the lacrimal sac. If the irrigant enters the nose heavily stained with fluorescein, the upper segment of the system is normal. If the irrigant enters the nose clear, the puncta and canaliculi are faulty. If no fluid is recovered from the nose, there is a complete obstruction.

Dacrocystogram (DCG)

This is similar to sac wash-out, except that instead of saline, a radiopaque dye is used and X-ray pictures are taken.

Clinically, sac wash-out is most commonly used to assess patency of the naso-lacrimal system. It is only necessary to carry out Jones dye tests and DCG if surgery is considered. In fact, many surgeons would not normally perform these tests even before surgery.

Management of dry eyes and watery eyes

Dry eye syndrome is commonly associated with lid margin disease such as blepharitis and Meibomian gland dysfunction. It is important to treat these associated conditions. A mucolytic agent is occasionally required if there is excessive mucus production. Otherwise, patients should be given tear supplements to be used as often as they wish. It is vital to reassure the patients that lack of tears will not damage their eyes.

Watery eyes in the elderly are commonly caused by medial ectropion or by the blockage of the naso-lacrimal system. It is, however, important to exclude causes of increased tear production such as allergic reaction and excessive reflex secretion in dry eyes. Medial ectropion can be corrected by a simple lid operation.

Dacrocystorhinotomy (DCR) can be used to clear blockage of the naso-lacrimal system. It is, however, a relatively major operation which often requires general anaesthesia with variable success rate. Therefore, it is generally not recommended. As with dry eyes, it is equally important to reassure the patients that watery eyes would not damage their eyes. New techniques, such as laser rhinotomy and balloon dilatation of the naso-lacrimal duct, are under investigation, and may in the future become more acceptable options.

Chapter 3

Cornea and sclera

The cornea is an unusual structure in the human body. It is multilayered, yet it is transparent. Traditionally, transparency is the most important physiological property of the cornea.

With advances in ophthalmology, many other properties of the cornea have been studied. In recent years, the advances of keratorefractive surgery, in particular the use of the excimer laser to correct refractive errors, opens a new area of research in corneal healing.

Our understanding of corneal properties also improves our understanding of ocular penetration of topical ophthalmic preparations. The concept of the cornea being a privileged site for transplantational surgery has also been challenged. This will be discussed further in the chapter on immunology.

Corneal anatomy

The cornea is traditionally divided into five layers:

- Epithelium.
- Bowman's membrane.
- Stroma.
- Descemet's membrane.
- Endothelium.

It is now understood that there is a thin basement membrane under the epithelium and the Bowman's membrane is, in fact, modified superficial stroma.

Biochemistry of the cornea

Epithelium

- High activities of enzymes of glycolysis, Kreb's cycle and ATPase pump.
- High concentration of acetylcholine and cholinesterases — uncertain role.

Stroma

- Corneal fibrils are neatly organized.
- Typical 64–66 nm periodicity of collagen.
- Collagen similar to tendon and skin collagen.
- High in nitrogen, glycine, proline and hydroxyproline content.
- Glycosaminoglycans (GAG) occupy the interfibrillar space.
- GAG is believed to play a major role in the maintenance of corneal transparency.
- Low enzymatic activities.

Descemet's membrane

- Consists of type IV collagen (basement membrane type collagen).
- High glycine, hydroxyglycine and hydroxyproline content.
- Glycoproteins are tightly bound to the protein moiety.
- Highly elastic and forms a barrier.

Electrolyte composition of the cornea

The electrolyte composition of the cornea is summarized in Table 3.1.

Table 3.1 Electrolyte composition of the cornea (mmol/l)

	Na^+	K^+	CL^-
Whole cornea	156	28	97
Corneal stroma	172	21	108
Corneal epithelium	75	142	30
Aqueous humour	143	5	108
Plasma	151	5	109

Transparency of the cornea

The normal cornea is transparent; this is enabled because of the regular arrangement of the stromal collagen fibrils and the relative corneal dehydration.

Physical properties required to maintain transparency

- Corneal collagen fibrils form a lattice structure.
- The scattering of light is eliminated by mutual interference from individual fibrils, hence the cornea appears clear.
- Any interference to this structure, including swelling, would increase light scatter and the cornea appears hazy.
- The cornea is also avascular.

Corneal dehydration

The normal cornea maintains a reasonably constant water content at about 75–80% of its weight. Clinically, increase in hydration results in increase of thickness and reduction of transparency of the cornea.

This relative dehydration can be influenced by the following factors:

- Anatomic integrity of endothelium and epithelium.
- Electrolyte and osmotic balances.
- Metabolic activities.
- Evaporation of water through the anterior surface.
- Intraocular pressure.

Integrity of both the endothelium and the epithelium seems to be important to maintain corneal transparency. The endothelium actively removes fluid from the stroma through the Na-K ATPase pump. There is also evidence that the epithelium has a chloride pump stimulated by adrenaline and cyclic AMP.

Evaporation of water increases the osmolarity of the tear film. This hypertonicity would draw water from the cornea and maintain cornea dehydration. Clinically, glycerine is used temporarily to clear a swollen cornea by increasing the osmolarity of the tear film.

A rise in intraocular pressure to over 50 mmHg often results in corneal oedema. It is believed that the high intraocular pressure compromises endothelial cell function and hence reduces the ability of the cornea to remain relatively dehydrated.

Corneal wound healing

Epithelial healing

Small defects

- Nearby epithelial cells retract and become round shaped initially.
- They begin an amoeboid sliding movement to the exposed defect and form a new monolayer of cells.
- These cells then take the role as the new basal layer and undergo mitosis.
- The defect is filled with the normal four to five layers of cells.
- Most small defects would be healed within 24–48 hours.

Large defects

- Total loss of corneal epithelium is not uncommon following many corneal surgical procedures and chemical injuries.
- The limbal conjunctival cells move across the basement membrane and undergo mitosis as corneal epithelial cells in smaller defects.
- Mucous glands and melanocytes may be brought along with the cellular migration, however, the new corneal epithelial cells become quite typical in appearance and lose the conjunctival properties very rapidly.

- It would take a few days to form a monolayer of cells and several weeks before firm desmosomal attachment established between the newly formed basal epithelial cells and the basement membrane.

Clinical points

Fluorescein is used to detect corneal epithelial defects. Penetration of fluorescein into the corneal epithelium is normally excluded by the tight intercellular junction of the surface epithelial cells. When these junctions are disrupted, as in corneal abrasion or ulcer, the dye can pass through the basement membrane rapidly and stains the anterior stroma, leaving an easily visible green mark on the corneal surface.

The constant blinking action of the upper eyelid tends to scrap off the new cells as they move across the basement membrane. Therefore, it has been usual to immobilize the lid by applying an eye pad in patients with a corneal abrasion. Recent studies have not shown any significant clinical differences whether an eye pad is used or not for simple corneal abrasion. For total or subtotal epithelial defects, immobilization of the upper lid by a temporary tarsorrhaphy using either sutures or Botulinum toxin makes a significant difference in the overall healing time.

Until the firm desmosomal attachment between the newly formed basal epithelial cells and the basement membrane is established, the corneal epithelium can be lifted easily by oedema fluid or by attachment to the posterior surface of the upper eyelid during sleep. The latter can give rise to the condition called recurrent erosion, when the patient presents with painful red eye in the morning even months after a minor corneal injury. This is treated by nocturnal application of simple eye ointment to lubricate the eye during sleep, hence reducing the attachment between the corneal epithelium and the upper lid.

In chemical injuries, the limbal conjunctival cells can also be damaged. It is important to assess for limbal ischaemia and necrosis in these situations. Limbal conjunctival autograft surgery by taking conjunctival graft tissue from the other eye to promote corneal healing may be required.

Stromal healing

- Laceration of the stroma causes rapid accumulation of extracellular fluid on either side of the wound from the water and electrolytes of the tear film.

- Keratocytes retract their processes and take on the features of fibroblasts.
- Polymorphonuclear leucocytes and monocytes enter the wound through tear film or limbal arcades if the wound is close to the limbus.
- Monocytes also begin to take the appearance of fibroblasts.
- Procollagen is formed by these modified keratocytes and monocytes.
- The epithelium might be healed at this stage and in fact might completely fill the wound to the corneal surface.
- Procollagen matures rapidly into collagen.
- The acute inflammatory response is reduced and less cellular component remains.
- Strengthening and remodeling of the area occur.
- Epithelium that has entered the stroma is gradually forced out until only a small facet remains.
- Irregular collagen fibrils and corneal lamellae in the stroma beneath the facet persist.
- Due to this irregularity, healed corneal wounds are almost invariably opaque.
- This opacity may be very thin if the wound was not gaping widely, as in the surgical incision for cataract surgery.
- The original corneal tensile strength takes months to return.

Descemet's membrane and endothelium healing

- The Descemet's membrane splits and curls away from the wound margin.
- The nearby endothelial cells begin to enlarge and cover the defect by amoeboid movement.
- These cells secrete a new layer of Descemet's membrane.
- The curled edges of the Descemet's membrane often remain, although they are covered in part by the new membrane and appear clinically as Descemet's folds.
- The overlying stroma is often oedematous in the repair stage, indicating endothelium pump failure.
- The endothelial cells do not have mitotic ability; if the damage is extensive, the cornea may become permanently swollen.

Full thickness laceration

- The wound is usually plugged by fibrin and iris tissue presenting as iris prolapse.
- This tissue undergoes fibrosis and scar formation if repair is not carried out.
- The wound is often vascularized by the iris stroma.

Clinical points

The original corneal tensile strength in a penetrating corneal graft might take a few years, if ever, to return to normal. Topical steroids, which are essential for graft survival, can also decrease the rate of wound healing and hence reduce wound strength.

In photorefractive keratoplasty (PRK), the conventional excimer laser technique for refractive errors, the epithelium is scraped off mechanically. The laser is then applied to the corneal stroma to remodel the corneal shape in achieving the desirable refractive correction. The main problem is the combined corneal epithelial and stromal healing process leading to opacity formation. Theoretically, topical steroids can be used to reduce the healing process and hence scarring. Nonetheless, no significant clinical benefit has been found.

Other techniques are being developed to overcome this problem. In laser in situ keratomileusis (LASIK), an anterior corneal flap of about 0.1–0.2 mm thick is created and hinged up, and the stromal bed is then remodelled by laser. After laser treatment, the corneal flap is replaced and as the flap is so thin, suturing is usually not required. The preservation of the epithelium and the Bowman's membrane accelerates the wound healing process. The early results are very encouraging and significant opacity is uncommon.

Corneal penetration of topical medications

Medications required to penetrate the cornea should be able to diffuse through the high lipid content corneal epithelial and endothelial cells as well as the high water content stroma. Ionized solutions penetrate poorly through the lipid-rich epithelium and endothelium but quickly through the stroma. The reverse is true for fat-soluble compounds.

Hence, the medication should exist in both ionized and non-ionized forms. The non-ionized form would penetrate the epithelium, become ionized in the stroma, return to non-ionized form in the endothelium, becoming ionized once again in the anterior chamber.

Surface active agents which increase the wetting effect of drugs appear to enhance corneal permeability by disrupting the epithelial barrier, allowing drugs to penetrate between the cells of the corneal epithelium.

Contact time between the drug and the cornea can be raised by increasing the viscosity of the drug solution. This can favour penetration. That is also how gel and ointment preparations result in better penetration.

Sclera

- The sclera is composed of extracellular tissue in the form of collagen and mucopolysaccharide.
- Tough, opaque and mainly avascular.
- Unlike the cornea, collagen is not organized in an orderly fashion and there is no clearly defined epithelium and endothelium.
- Despite that, if the sclera is allowed to dehydrate, it becomes translucent.
- The Tenon's capsule is a fibrous tissue which surrounds the sclera.
- The blood and nerve supply enter the sclera through a fine layer of episcleral tissue which lies just under the Tenon.

Scleral rigidity

- The sclera is under constant pressure from the intraocular pressure.
- It maintains the stable viscoelastic structure of the eye.
- It stretches proportionately more with initial elevations of intraocular pressure.
- As the pressure increases, the resistance to further stretching also increases.
- Hence a small increase in intraocular volume at low pressure, allowing for more stretching, results in a small increase in intraocular pressure.

- However, at high pressure, the same increase of intraocular volume would result in a larger increase in intraocular pressure as stretching resistance increases.
- This is defined as the scleral rigidity.

Clinical points

- Abnormal scleral rigidity is associated with high myopia, inflammatory diseases and previous conventional retinal detachment surgery.
- It was important in the past as the intraocular pressure measurement by the indentation method increases the intraocular volume significantly and hence can give a false reading.
- Using the modern applanation method, the intraocular volume does not alter significantly (see Chapter 4).

Chapter 4

Aqueous humour and intraocular pressure

Outline

Control of intraocular pressure
Measurement of intraocular pressure
    Fixed-force tonometer
        Maklakoff tonometer
        Posner–Inglima tonometer
    Fixed-area tonometer
        Goldmann tonometer
        Perkins tonometer
        Non-contact air puff tonometer
    Indentation tonometer
        Schiotz tonometer

The aqueous humour is a clear watery solution secreted by the ciliary processes into the posterior chamber of the eye. It circulates to the anterior chamber through the pupil. As it bathes the lens and cornea, there is an exchange of nutrients and waste. Most of the aqueous leaves the eye through the trabecular meshwork into the Schlemm's canal and the episcleral venous system.

This circulation maintains an intraocular pressure (IOP) in the eye which is higher than the atmospheric pressure. This prevents the collapse of the eye. The equilibrium of aqueous formation and outflow rates is of crucial importance. If the latter is reduced significantly, the IOP rises, which in turn can cause ganglion cell damage in the retina. This plays a role in the condition called glaucoma which affects about 1.5–2% of the population in their lifetime.

Functions of aqueous

- Carries oxygen and nutrient to the lens and cornea.
- Carries waste products away from lens and cornea.
- Maintains the shape and internal structure of the eye by sustaining an intraocular pressure higher than atmospheric pressure.
- Flushes away blood, macrophages and other inflammatory cells and products from the anterior chamber.

Formation of aqueous

The ciliary processes are responsible for the formation of aqueous under the influence of β-adrenergic receptors. Three inter-dependent physiological systems are believed to be involved in the formation and chemical composition of the aqueous.

- Diffusion.
- Dialysis and ultrafiltration.
- Active secretion.

Diffusion

Basic principles of diffusion

- Molecules in a fluid medium (air or liquid) are in constant, random motion.
- When there is an uneven distribution of molecules in the medium, the molecules will move from the higher concentrated areas to the lower concentrated area; this is called a diffusion gradient.
- This is also true when the two areas are separated by a membrane; as long as this membrane is permeable to the molecule or particle concerned, then the diffusion gradient will develop.
- An equilibrium will be achieved when the concentrations of the particle concerned are the same on each side of the membrane.
- At equilibrium, movement across the membrane still occurs; however, the number of particles going in one direction equals the number going the other way, hence there is no net movement.
- It should be noted that water participates in this process as well, the net movement of water usually being opposite to the movement of the particles (solute).

Fick's law of diffusion

Rate of movement = K (C1–C2)

where K = constant
          C1 = Concentration on the side with higher
                  concentration
          C2 = Concentration on the side with lower
                  concentration

The K constant is low (i.e. lower rate of movement) if there is:

- Low membrane permeability.

- Low temperature.
- High viscosity of the fluid medium.

Therefore, diffusion tends to occur more rapidly in extra-cellular fluids than across cells. However, in the ciliary processes, it is a dynamic system. The environment changes rapidly due to other co-existing factors. Diffusion should be seen as one of such factors in this dynamic process.

Dialysis and ultrafiltration

Basic principles of dialysis

- In most biological solutions, there is a combination of small molecules, such as salt and glucose, and larger molecules, such as plasma proteins.
- Most cellular membranes will allow free movements of small molecules and water but not the plasma proteins.
- So, if a solution of salt and protein is separated from a less concentrated salt solution, there will be a net movement of water to the protein side and opposite net movement of salt by diffusion.
- This is called dialysis, and can be used to remove unwanted salts in a physiological system.

Basic principles of ultrafiltration

- The exchange of salt and water can be accelerated by adding a hydrostatic pressure on the protein-rich side of the membrane.
- This is called ultrafiltration.
- The rate of movement is higher and the final concentration of salt might be slightly different.
- This process occurs, for instance, in capillary walls, where there is higher pressure and protein concentration in plasma as compared with the extracellular space.

Gibbs–Donnan effect

- As the protein usually carries an electrical charge (usually negative), the positive ions will tend to be bound to the protein; thus there would be an excess of sodium and potassium on the protein side.

- This is called the Gibbs–Donnan effect.
- In order to maintain electrical balance, the total positive (sodium and potassium ions) and negative charges (protein, chloride ions and other negative charged ions) must be equal on both sides of the membrane.
- So, if the formation of aqueous is by ultrafiltration alone under the Gibbs–Donnan effect, the aqueous should be a protein-free solution with less sodium and potassium than plasma and more chloride and bicarbonate than plasma.
- That is not the case in aqueous humour; hence, active secretion occurs (*vide infra*).

Active secretion

- Active secretion implies an energy consuming process to transport substances across cell membrane against a diffusion gradient.
- In the ciliary epithelium, the sodium pump is mainly mediated by the enzyme system called sodium-potassium activated adenosine triphosphatase (Na-K ATPase).
- Sodium is pumped across the cell membrane whilst chloride ion and water are passively carried through to maintain the electrical and concentration equilibrium.
- The system is powered by the citric acid cycle.
- The role of carbonic anhydrase in aqueous formation is still unknown.
- It is believed that the enzyme acts as a facilitator or catalyst for the Na-K ATPase system; it could also be a related parallel process or the enzyme may maintain an optimal environment (such as pH) for the Na-K ATPase system.
- Its inhibition significantly reduces the formation of aqueous.

Physiological processes in the ciliary body

- Active cellular secretion which requires energy.
- Sodium, potassium, ascorbate and bicarbonate are transported from plasma to the posterior chamber.
- Chloride and water follow through passively to maintain electrical and concentration equilibrium.

- Amino acids and other substances are also actively transported.
- Other small molecules cross the membrane in the aqueous, probably by diffusion and ultrafiltration.
- Prostaglandins and some other drugs and substances can be actively transported out of the eye. It is believed that this physiological mechanism provides a mean to remove potentially harmful material out of the eye.

Physical properties and composition of aqueous

- Anterior and posterior chamber volumes are about 0.25 ml and 0.06 ml, respectively.
- Refractive index of 1.3336 which is lower than that of cornea; hence light diverges slightly in the cornea–aqueous interface.
- Viscosity and density are slightly higher than water.
- Osmolarity is slightly higher than plasma.
- Very low protein concentration — 0.2 % of the concentration of plasma proteins.
- Amino acids concentrations are higher than that of plasma.
- Hydrogen and chloride ion concentrations are also higher.
- Bicarbonate ions concentration is lower.
- Sodium ions concentration is similar to that of plasma.
- Ascorbate and lactate concentrations are much higher.
- Glucose, urea and nonproteinous nitrogen concentrations are slightly lower.

Blood–aqueous barrier

Large molecules such as plasma proteins do not get into the aqueous even when the plasma concentration is very high. This is commonly referred as the blood–aqueous barrier.

The sites of this barrier are most likely to be in the tight junctions between the epithelial cells and in the basement membrane. The barrier is not absolute; medium size and water soluble substance may penetrate but usually at a slower rate than passing through capillary walls.

Breakdown of the blood–aqueous barrier

The blood–aqueous barrier is fragile and can be easily broken down by various mechanisms, including:

- Intraocular surgery.
- Corneal abrasion.
- Blunt trauma.
- Intraocular inflammation.
- Vascular dilatation secondary excessive histamine production.
- Anterior segment ischaemia.
- X-ray and β-radiation.
- Alkali and other irritants.
- Cholinergic drugs such as pilocarpine.
- Cholinesterase inhibitors such as ecothiopate.

When the blood–aqueous barrier is broken down, inflammatory cells and even fibrin can be present in the aqueous, which can be seen clinically in slit-lamp microscopy examinations. It is generally believed that prostaglandin release plays a major role in the final pathway of this process.

Factors affecting aqueous formation rate

The aqueous formation rate is not constant and it seems to have a diurnal cycle. There are a number of factors which increase and decrease its formation. Although a decrease of aqueous formation is usually associated with a reduction of intraocular pressure (IOP), it is not necessarily always the case. For instance, aqueous formation rate decreases with age but the IOP increases with age as the aqueous outflow rate also decreases with age and to a larger extent than the former.

Factors that reduce aqueous formation rate

- Age.
- Exercise.
- Reduced blood pressure — decreases ciliary body blood flow.
- Hypothermia — reduces metabolic rate and hence active secretion.

- Increased intraocular pressure — decreases ciliary body blood flow.
- Anterior segment inflammation.
- Retinal detachment — ciliary body shut-down.
- Choroidal detachment — ciliary body shut-down.
- Cyclodialysis — ciliary body shut-down.
- Adrenalectomy — through hormonal effects.
- Carbonic anhydrase inhibitors — commonly used anti-glaucoma therapy.
- β-Adrenergic receptor blockers — commonly used anti-glaucoma therapy.
- Cannabis — ongoing research in finding a topical preparation.
- Spironolactone and cardiac glycoside — effect too small for therapeutic use.
- Retrobulbar and peribulbar anaesthesia — reduces simulation from ciliary ganglion.
- Cyclodestruction therapy — damages the ciliary body by cryotherapy or laser.

Factors that increase aqueous formation rate

- Reduced plasma osmolality (by drinking large quantities of water) — increases the osmotic force in the ciliary epithelium.
- Adrenaline — stimulates β-adrenergic receptors in the ciliary epithelium. (It was believed in the past that adrenaline reduces aqueous formation; some ophthalmologists still use adrenaline as anti-glaucoma therapy; the mode of action is, however, to increase aqueous outflow.)

Aqueous pathway within the eye

- The aqueous is secreted by the ciliary processes into the posterior chamber.
- It would pass through the pupil into the anterior chamber without any hindrance.
- Most of the aqueous leaves the eye through the trabecular meshwork or the uveoscleral pathway.

Aqueous movement in the anterior chamber

- The hydrostatic force directs the aqueous from the pupillary margin peripherally to the drainage angle.
- As the more posterior aqueous is nearer to the warm iris, it is carried upward whilst the anterior aqueous near to the cooler cornea is carried downward. It forms a convection current which is commonly seen in slit-lamp examination of patients with iritis by the movement of inflammatory cells.
- Gravity also tends to carry pigment, blood and debris to the inferior angle.

Aqueous outflow

There are two main outflow mechanisms:

- The conventional outflow through the trabecular meshwork into the Schlemm's canal and the episcleral vessels (75–80%).
- The uveoscleral pathway through the anterior face of the ciliary body into the choroidal vessels (20–25%).

Conventional pathway

- The main aqueous outflow resistance seems to be in the junction of the outer corneoscleral trabecular spaces and the Schlemm's canal, which is believed to have a valvular action controlled by the ciliary muscle activity.
- Outflow resistance increases with ciliary muscle relaxation which can be induced pharmacologically by using atropine-like anticholinergic drugs.
- The reverse is also true; accommodation and cholinergic activities decrease resistance, which can be induced by mitotics like pilocarpine, used in the treatment of glaucoma.
- Large particles and cells are compressed and deformed in the trabecular meshwork before leaving the eye.
- Phagocytosis by endothelial cells plays only a minor role in the removal of these cells and debris.

Uveoscleral pathway

- This pathway is independent of intraocular pressure changes.
- It handles about 0.5 µl/min.

- It is decreased by miotics and increased by cycloplegic agents (the reverse of the conventional pathway).
- This is because miotics cause ciliary muscle contraction, which closes the gap in the ciliary muscle bundles and prevents aqueous outflow.
- Prostaglandin and α_2-adrenergic receptor agonists increase outflow in this pathway significantly, but the exact mechanism is unknown.

Clinical points

Pathophysiology of acute glaucoma

- Normally, the aqueous would pass through the pupil into the anterior chamber without any hindrance.
- The pressure difference between the posterior and anterior chambers is very small.
- If the flow is restricted by any blockage in the pupillary region, the pressure in the posterior chamber can build up very quickly.
- The peripheral iris can bow forward causing iris bombé.
- The iris then blocks the outflow channels and the pressure of the eye rises very quickly.
- This process is believed to be the pathophysiology of acute angle closure glaucoma.

Intraocular pressure (IOP)

- The average IOP is about 15 mmHg.
- The range of IOP is between 8 and 21 mmHg.
- Diurnal variation is present; it is traditionally believed that it is highest in the morning (8 a.m.) and lowest in late evening (8 p.m.). Some recent studies suggested that it is highest at about 12 p.m. and lowest at 2 a.m.
- The diurnal pattern might be associated with plasma corticosteroid concentration but this has never been proven.
- Seasonal variation occurs, highest in winter and lowest in summer.

Mathematical expression of IOP

- Fluids flow if there is a pressure difference.
- From high pressure to low pressure.
- In the eye, the flow can be expressed mathematically.

Flow = (IOP–EVP) × C

By rearranging the formula

IOP = Flow/C + EVP or IOP = Flow × R + EVP

IOP = Intraocular pressure
EVP = Episcleral venous pressure
R = Resistance of outflow
C = Facility of outflow (the reciprocal of resistance)

In other words, any increase in flow, resistance of outflow or episcleral venous pressure will increase IOP and any decrease in any of these factors will reduce IOP.

Factors raising IOP

Increased episcleral venous pressure

- Large increase of blood pressure.
- Increase carotid blood flow.
- Increase central venous pressure.
- Valsalva manoeuvre.
- Carotid–cavernous fistula.
- Hypercarbia.
- Blockage of ophthalmic vein.
- Sturge–Weber syndrome.

Increase of flow

Any source of external pressure to the eye or hypersecretion of aqueous would increase flow:

- Co-contraction of extraocular muscles, e.g. in Duane's syndrome.
- Restricted extraocular muscles, e.g. in dysthyroid eye disease and blow-out fracture.
- Acute external pressure.

- Forced blinking.
- Succinylcholine — polarizing agent causes initial contraction of extraocular muscles.
- Plasma hypo-osmolality — water drinking increase aqueous formation.

Increase outflow resistance

- Age.
- Blockage of trabecular meshwork.
- Relaxation of accommodation.
- Cycloplegic agents.
- Corticosteroids — in steroid responder (see Pharmacology chapter).

Factors lowering IOP

Reduced episcleral venous pressure

- Large decrease of blood pressure.
- Decrease carotid blood flow.
- Decrease central venous pressure — by standing up.

Decrease of flow

Any reduction of aqueous formation would reduce flow:

- Retinal detachment — ciliary body shut-down.
- Choroidal detachment — ciliary body shut-down.
- Cyclodialysis — ciliary body shut-down.
- Adrenalectomy.
- Carbonic anhydrase inhibitors.
- β-Adrenergic receptor blockers.
- Cannabis.
- Spironolactone and cardiac glycoside.
- Retrobulbar and peribulbar anaesthesia.
- Cyclodestruction therapy.
- General and local anaesthesia — reduce muscle tone.

Decrease outflow resistance

- Adrenaline and related compound.
- Miotics.
- Prostaglandins — initial IOP rise is common.
- Ocular trauma — secondary to prostaglandins effect.
- Accommodation.

Control of IOP

- The intraocular pressure varies within a limited range; it has been suggested that some regulating mechanism exists.
- Some evidence of CNS involvement.
- When IOP is high, aqueous production decreases; this is called pseudofacility.
- β-Adrenergic receptors are presented in the ciliary body; it is now believed to increase aqueous formation and hence increase IOP if stimulated.
- α_2-Adrenergic receptors and prostaglandins seem to play a major role in the decrease of outflow resistance and hence reduce IOP.

Measurement of IOP

- The pressure inside a flexible sphere can be closely approximated by knowing the force required to flatten a given area.
- Under Imbert–Fick law, pressure = force/area.
- The pressure can be determined by measuring the force necessary to flatten a fixed area or by measuring the area flattened by a fixed force.

Fixed-force tonometer

Maklakoff tonometer

- First developed in 1855.
- A dye is smeared on the anaesthetized cornea.
- The flat-bottomed known weight is allowed to rest on the cornea.

- The dye is transferred from the flattened cornea to the tonometer bottom.
- The area of applanation can then be calculated from the diameter of the circle of dye on the tonometer bottom.
- As the weight is known, the pressure can be derived from the Imbert–Fick formula.
- The main problem is that a relatively large area of cornea is flattened by a relatively heavy weight, while a small amount of intraocular fluid is displaced.
- Thus the tonometer measures pressure in the eye with the tonometer on it rather than the true IOP.
- The true IOP can be calculated from the measured pressure by assuming all eyes respond to the tonometer in the same way.
- Other factors such as scleral rigidity can affect this calculation and cause error.
- Smeared ink secondary to eye and tonometer movement during measuring can also be the source of error.

Posner–Inglima tonometer

- It is based on the same principles of the Maklakoff tonometer.
- The only difference is that this tonometer is plastic and light-weighted, hence reduce displacement of ocular fluid.
- The error from other ocular factors is reduced.

Fixed-area tonometer

Goldmann tonometer

- This instrument is generally referred as the gold standard for IOP measurement in clinical settings.
- It is mounted on the slit-lamp.
- The applanating surface has a diameter of 3.06 mm placed in the centre of a plastic cylinder of 7 mm total diameter.
- The plastic cylinder is attached to an arm that ultimately is pushed forward by a spring-loaded knob.
- When the corneal surface is flattened by the plastic cylinder, the tear layer is squeezed out from the surface.

- Two prisms are placed in the plastic cylinder, apex to apex, so that the ring of the tear meniscus is optically converted into two half-rings.
- The prisms are so placed that the two half-rings, one above and one below, are separated by 3.06 mm (see Figure 4.1).
- The force required is small and hence very little displacement of intraocular fluid occurs.
- The corneal elasticity will push back the tonometer head and this force can cause overestimation of IOP.
- The surface tension and capillary attraction of the tear film would pull the tonometer head towards the cornea and hence underestimate IOP.
- These two forces would be balanced out when the applanating diameter is between 3 and 4 mm.
- At 3.06 mm, the force measured in grams can be converted to IOP in mmHg by simply multiplying the former by 10.
- If corneal astigmatism is over 3 diopters, the doubling prism needs to be turned 45 degrees from the axis of the astigmatism or else an error of 2–3 mmHg can be induced.
- Corneal scarring alters the corneal elasticity and causes under-estimation of IOP.

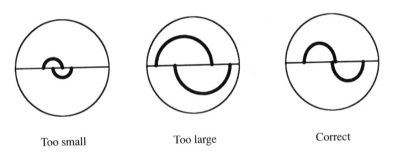

Too small   Too large   Correct

Figure 4.1 Tear meniscus arcs as seen in Goldmann applanation tonometer

Perkins tonometer

- This is a portable version of the Goldmann tonometer.
- The basic principles are the same.

Non-contact air puff tonometer

- This instrument is based on the principle of the Goldmann tonometer.
- A puff of air whose force increases linearly over 8 ms is directed at the cornea.
- It is designed so that it hits the cornea with a known, reproducible area.
- The air pulse then progressively flattens the cornea.
- An optical sensor is so positioned that an oblique light would be reflected into it when the cornea is flat and acting as a plane mirror.
- The air generator is switched off at that point.
- The computer can then calculate the force required and determine the IOP.
- The method correlates well with the Goldmann tonometer in normal IOP, but tends to overestimate in higher IOP.
- The system can be used without anaesthesia.

Indentation tonometer

Schiotz tonometer

- A known force will indent a fluid filled object to a greater degree if the internal pressure is high.
- The plunger in the Schiotz raises the intraocular pressure from its resting state to a value 50–100% higher when it is first placed in the eye (see Figure 4.2).

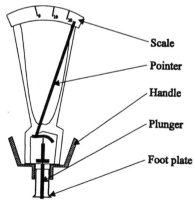

Scale

Pointer

Handle

Plunger

Foot plate

Figure 4.2 The Schiotz tonometer

- The plunger then pushes into the cornea until the eye pushes back.
- In a soft eye (low IOP), the plunger would sink more before it stops.
- The IOP can be calculated by knowing the scale reading and the plunger load.
- The Schiotz conversion table assumes an average scleral rigidity which can be a major source of errors.

It is cheap, portable and simple to use and maintain; nevertheless, its clinical use is restricted to when Goldmann or Perkins tonometers are not available.

Chapter 5

Crystalline lens

Outline

During cataract surgery, part of the anterior capsule can be peeled off. The epithelium, located immediately beneath the anterior capsule, generally comes away with the capsule. The nucleus can then be removed by manual expression or by ultrasonic energy as in phacoemulsification. The cortex which surrounds the nucleus is aspirated by suction. A capsular bag is remained for the positioning of an intraocular implant (Figure 5.1).

Composition of the lens

The lens is rather unusual in having a relatively low water content (65%) and a very high protein content (34%). The remaining solids (1%) include inorganic ions, organic phosphates, nucleic acids and metabolites.

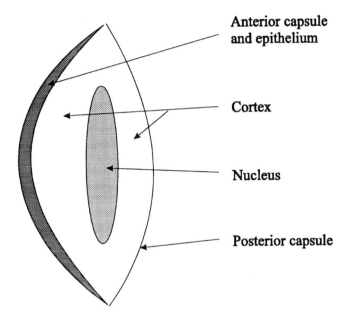

Figure 5.1 Anatomy of the lens

Lens water

- The overall water content is about 65% but the distribution varies.
- The capsule contains 80% water, lens cortex 68.6% and lens nucleus 63.4%.
- Normal human lens shows no significant alteration in hydration with age.
- The majority of lens water is 'free water', i.e. not protein bound.
- As the lens fibres are closely packed together, only a small portion of the lens water is located in the extracellular space.

Proteins

More than 85% of lens proteins are soluble. They are divided into α-crystallin, β-crystallin and γ-crystallin based on molecular weight in descending order. The insoluble lens protein is called the albuminoid.

α-*Crystallin*

- Molecular weight of 800,000 to 1 million.
- Comprised of 40–50 polypeptide chains.
- About 32% of total lens protein.
- More in the cortical region than the nucleus.
- It is suggested that albuminoid is derived from α-crystallin.

β-*Crystallin*

- Molecular weight of 50,000–500,000.
- About 54% of total lens protein.
- The properties of β-crystallin are poorly understood.

γ-*Crystallin*

- Molecular weight of about 20,000.
- About 1.5% of total lens protein.
- Mainly synthesized in embryonic lens.
- More in the nucleus than in the cortex.
- Some γ-crystallin fraction can inhibit mitosis in lens epithelium.

Albuminoid

- About 12.5% of total lens protein.
- Two major components.
- About 10% of albuminoid are lens fibre membrane.
- The remaining portion is probably converted from α-crystallin.
- The latter has almost identical amino acid composition and immunological properties to α-crystallin.
- More in the nucleus than cortex region.

Immunochemistry of lens protein

- Lens protein shows an organ specific immune reaction.
- If an animal is sensitized to lens protein of another animal, the animal would develop antibodies which react with antigens in lens extracted from almost all other species.

- This suggests that lens proteins are similar in different species.
- Interestingly, a patient can be sensitized by his own lens protein and will develop a phacoanaphylactic reaction.

Energy metabolism of the lens

- The main pathway for glucose metabolism in the lens is by anaerobic glycolysis.
- The rate limiting stage is on the conversion of glucose to glucose-6-phosphate by the enzyme hexokinase.
- About 80% of the glucose is converted to lactic acid, which diffuses out into the aqueous humour.
- Aerobic process would be more efficient; however, the lens has low oxygen tension.
- Only about 3% of glucose is metabolized through the Kreb's cycle (aerobic), yet it produces about 20% of the energy.
- Two other significant pathways in glucose metabolism are the sorbitol pathway and hexose monophosphate shunt (see Figure 5.2).
- The sorbitol pathway has a role in the development of sugar cataract (*vide infra*).

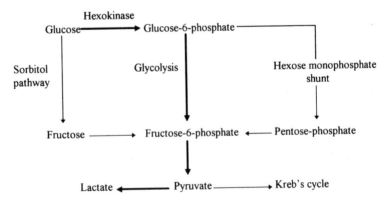

Figure 5.2 Major pathways of glucose metabolism in the lens. The thicker arrow indicates the normal pathway.

Clinical points

Pathophysiology of cataract

The lens is transparent; when any part of it becomes opaque, it is termed cataract. The incidence of cataract increases with age, and by the age of 70, most people would have some degree of cataract. Surgery is only required if there is visual impairment, although cataract surgery is the most commonly performed intraocular surgery. There are many observed causes of cataract, but the exact pathophysiology is still poorly understood.

Change in protein content

- With increasing age, there is an increase in the proportion of insoluble protein and an increase in total lens size as a result of continual growth.
- In cataractous lenses, the insoluble portion can be more than 35% as compared with 12.5% in normal lenses.
- It is believed that this is caused by the combination of a decrease in soluble protein and an increase in conversion of soluble to insoluble protein.
- Yellow colouration is common in the aging lens; this colouration provides an effective filter for harmful ultra-violet light.
- In nuclear sclerosis cataract, there is a significant increase of this colouration and it is believed that ultra-violet light plays a role in its occurrence.
- The pigment might be associated with the insoluble protein.

Chemical changes

- In nuclear cataract, there is no change in ion and water concentration.
- In cortical cataract, sodium concentration increases dramatically with decrease in potassium.
- Calcium level also increases with increased hydration.

Glutathione

- Glutathione has attracted research interest as it is markedly reduced in cataractous lenses.

- It is a tripeptide made up of glycine, cysteine and glutamic acid.
- There is a very high glutathione concentration in the lens.
- Most of it is presented in the reduced form (GSH).
- It is mostly synthesized within the lens, although active transport occurs.
- It was believed that glutathione maintains lens protein sulphydryl groups in the reduced state, which is essential for lens transparency. However, the evidence of this role for glutathione is uncertain.
- It is, however, a co-enzyme for a number of reaction and it also plays a role in a number of oxidation–reduction systems.
- The exact reason for its occurrence in reduced amounts in cataractous lenses is unknown.

Sugar cataract

- In diabetes mellitus, glucose levels in the aqueous increases, and thus more glucose enters the lens.
- The limited amount of hexokinase restricts glucose metabolism through glycolysis and hexose monophosphate shunt.
- The excess glucose is therefore shunted into the sorbitol pathway and is converted into sorbitol and fructose.
- The abnormally high concentration of sorbitol and fructose pulls water into the lens in order to maintain osmotic equilibrium.
- Cell swelling leads to cell rupture and the release of amino acids, potassium and so on; cataract develops.
- In galactosaemia (an inborn error of metabolism), galactose is converted into dulcitol by the aldose reductase in the sorbitol pathway.
- Dulcitol is unable to diffuse out of the lens cells and it cannot be metabolized.
- The high level of dulcitol causes rapid cataract formation by a similar mechanism to that mentioned above.

Radiation cataract

- Radiation damage involves primarily the germinative epithelial cells.
- It appears to cause an increase in lens membrane permeability.
- It can also affect cell division, protein metabolism and protein synthesis.
- Glutathione and RNA metabolism may also be affected.

The initial lens changes are seen in the posterior pole, followed by cortical involvement.

Refractive errors and emmetropization

Refractive errors occur when focal plane is not on the retina. If it is behind the retina, it is called hypermetropia, whilst that in front is called myopia. More people are, however, emmetropic (no refractive error) than would be expected.

An active emmetropization mechanism might guide the postnatal development of the eye, matching the axial length to the focal plane. The axial length initially is generally short so that the focal plane of the unaccommodated eye is behind the retina. Hence, hypermetropia is common in infancy. The subsequent axial elongation eventually align the retina to, but not past, the focal plane. When animals are raised with the focal plane shifted posteriorly with minus-power lenses, the eyes elongate to match the displaced focal plane.

In visual deprivation, the eyes elongate past the point of emmetropia and become myopic. It is suggested that the axial length is regulated within the eye itself, involving direct, spatially local communication from the retina to the sclera.

Chapter 6

Vitreous humour

The vitreous body occupies 80% of the entire volume of the eye. It is a clear gel containing 99% water; the remaining 1% comprises collagen, soluble proteins and hyaluronic acid. It is one of the simplest connective tissues and basically has no structure at all.

In the past, vitreous had not been examined extensively. With the advent of vitreoretinal surgery, it is now known that vitreous plays an important role in the pathophysiology of a number of vitreoretinal conditions. By removing the vitreous (vitrectomy), traction between the vitreous and retina is diminished. This becomes a standard treatment modality for a variety of vitreo-retinal diseases.

Biochemical properties

Collagen

- The fibrous protein in the vitreous is called vitrosin.
- Vitrosin differs from normal collagen in that 4–9% of its weight is a complex polysaccharide that cannot be separated from it.
- Nevertheless, it is most similar to type II collagen.

- It is believed that unlike other collagen, it is not a product of connective tissue cells, but rather of neuroectoderm origin.
- Vitrosin is most concentrated in the anterior portion of the vitreous body, particularly adjacent to the ciliary body, including the vitreous base. The concentration decreases toward the centre and posterior portions of the eye, but it becomes more concentrated near the retinal surface.
- The total collagen content increases from birth to adult life but no increase in concentration of collagen in vitreous occurs.

Soluble protein

- There is no significant synthesis or constant supply from the retina or the uveal tract.
- The soluble protein present at birth decreases to a negligible amount once the retinal vascularization process is completed.
- It is believed that these protein are important in the process of normal retinal vascularization and neovascularization.
- They are found in highest concentrations in the epiretinal cortical layer and lowest in the vitreous base (exact opposite to collagen concentration).
- The most abundant soluble proteins are vitreous globulin and albumin.
- Vitreous globulin consists largely of glycoproteins which are acidic in nature and have a high percentage of carbohydrate.

Hyaluronic acid

- This is a glycoaminoglycan with a molecular weight between 1 and 2 million.
- It is composed of N-acetyl-glucosamine and glucuronic acid in equal amounts.
- It occurs in the vitreous gel as soluble hyaluronate.
- The highly charged hydrated polysaccharide chain occupies a volume 1000 times greater than the chain would occupy in close packing.
- This hydrophilic substance forms a three-dimensional network intertwined amongst the collagen fibres.
- The hyaluronic chain adds the physical property of viscosity to the elasticity of the collagen network.

- The concentration is highest in the posterior cortex and lowest in the anterior periphery.
- It is believed that it is produced by hyalocytes within the vitreous.

Electrolytes

- The concentration of sodium is lower in the vitreous than in aqueous or plasma.
- Sodium enters the vitreous at its base via the posterior chamber and ciliary body.
- The turnover of sodium is slow and the outflow is through the anterior chamber.
- The potassium concentration is similar to that in aqueous but higher than plasma.
- There is an active carrier mechanism in the ciliary epithelium for potassium.
- There is also an active accumulation of potassium by the lens and a passive diffusion of potassium into the anterior vitreous occurs.
- Potassium leaves the vitreous mainly across the retina.
- Exchange of chloride occurs across the retina and posterior chamber.
- The concentration of chloride is higher in vitreous than aqueous and plasma.
- Bicarbonate enters the eye through the ciliary body.
- The concentration of bicarbonate is lower in vitreous than aqueous and plasma.
- The concentration of calcium in vitreous is similar to that in aqueous and plasma.

Glucose

- Glucose concentration is approximately half that of aqueous and plasma.
- Its main function is to maintain the metabolism of vitreous cells as well as the bordering tissues such as lens and retina.
- It enters the vitreous by diffusion through the retinal and choroidal circulation and ciliary body via the posterior chamber.

Physical properties

- The vitreous weighs about 4 g and its volume is about 4 ml.
- Water content is very high at about 99%.
- The density is between 1.0053 and 1.0089.
- The pH is about 7.5.
- The refractive index is 1.3347 which is very similar to that of aqueous.
- It transmits more than 90% of light between 350 and 800 nm; no transmission occurs beyond the 300 and 1400 nm limits.
- The vitreous–blood barrier prevents inflow of protein and hence maintain transparency.

Clinical points

Pathophysiology of posterior vitreous detachment (PVD)

Acute posterior vitreous detachment is a very common condition. In several studies in patients over 65 years of age, PVD is present in over 70%. In some cases, the patient presents with sudden onset of flashing lights and persistent vitreous floaters which is commonly described as spiders' webs, flies or rings. Nevertheless, in many cases, the event passes without any symptoms. It is important to examine the retina carefully in acute PVD, as it is associated with retinal tears.

- Threadlike demarcation of the vitreous fibrils starts in the around 45 years of age (earlier for myopes).
- Liquid-filled pockets called syneresis cavities are formed.
- These cavities enlarge and become confluent.
- Cortical vitreous degenerates and can enter into an acute phase.
- The thin remaining coat of cortical vitreous breaks suddenly.
- The collected fluid in the syneresis cavities empties itself into the preretinal space between the vitreous and retina.
- The condensed and collapsed vitreous is now found behind the lens and at the bottom of the vitreous cavity.
- A large optically empty retrovitreal space is formed.

- Glial tissue surrounding the optic disc forms a ring-shaped opacity which can be seen clinically as floaters; this ring is known as the Weiss ring.
- At this point, the clinical symptoms of flashing lights and floaters occur.
- Retinal tears can be formed by vitreous pull at places where the vitreous does not detach easily from the retina.
- Vitreous haemorrhage might follow such retinal damage; however, PVD on its own occasionally causes vitreous haemorrhage.

Vitreous opacities

The vitreous is normally clear and transparent, but it can be made opaque by blood, inflammatory cells and calcium soaps. Vitreous haemorrhage is possibly the most common cause of vitreous opacities. It is usually caused by proliferative diabetic retinopathy, retinal tears, blunt trauma and age-related maculopathy.

In posterior uveitis and endophthalmitis, inflammatory cells can pack the vitreous leading to so called 'vitritis'. In fact, the vitreous itself is not inflamed but the inflammatory cells get into the vitreous from surrounding inflamed tissues.

Asteroid hyalosis is a condition where white crystalline deposits are floating in the vitreous. It is surprising that it rarely causes any symptoms, although it can obscure the retina during fundal examination. The deposits are calcium soaps, which are usually bilateral and appear in the over-60s.

Pathological membranes in the vitreous

Three types of membranes can be found in the vitreous. The most common one is the epiretinal membrane (ERM), which is usually idiopathic but can be associated with diabetes and inflammatory eye diseases.

Membranes are also seen in patients with proliferative diabetic retinopathy (PDR) and proliferative vitreoretinopathy (PVR). It is believed that in both cases, the membranes are, in fact, scar tissue formation secondary to the insult to the eye. In PDR, new vessels are present; these vessels are supported by a fibrous tissue network. PDR membranes are usually more vascular, implying that they might originate from the fibrous network which has supported the neovascularization. These membranes can pull the retina and cause tractional retinal detachment.

In retinal detachment surgery, cryotherapy or laser therapy are used to induce adhesion between the retina and the choroid. These therapies or the surgery itself might induce an inflammatory response leading the formation of PVR. The origin of PVR membranes is unknown. It is believed that retinal pigment epithelial (RPE) cells play a role in its formation. Again, these membranes cause tractional retinal detachment. PVR formation remains the main obstacle for surgical success of retinal detachment surgery.

Chapter 7

Ocular circulation

The ophthalmic artery branches into the central retinal artery, two to three posterior ciliary arteries (PCAs) and several anterior ciliary arteries (ACAs). These vessels branch into two separate but inter-dependent vascular systems.

Anatomical considerations

Retinal vessels

- Branches of the central retinal artery (CRA).
- Arteries and veins are located within the nerve fibre layer distributed within the inner two thirds of the retina.

- The outer layers of the retina, includes the photoreceptors are nourished by the choroid.
- An avascular zone is seen centrally in the fovea (to reduce interference).
- The retinal capillaries are arranged in a laminated fashion with 2–3 layers of flat networks.
- The venous blood is drained by the central retinal vein which in turn drains into the cavernous sinus.
- The retrolaminar part of the optic nerve is supplied by the central retinal artery and pial vessels.

Uveal and ciliary vessels

- Branches of the posterior and anterior ciliary arteries (PCAs and ACAs).
- PCAs branch behind the globe into 10–20 short PCAs and two long PCAs.
- The short PCAs penetrate the sclera to supply the choriocapillaris.
- The long PCAs supply a sector of the nasal and temporal periphery of the choroid.
- The choriocapillaris is arranged in a lobular fashion with alternating feeding and draining vessels in the posterior pole, but becomes more spindle shaped patterns in the periphery.
- Choroidal blood drains into the vortex veins.
- There is usually one vortex vein in each quadrant of the posterior pole.
- The ACAs supply the anterior uvea which includes the iris, ciliary processes, ciliary body and the far peripheral choroid.
- Blood from the anterior uvea drains mainly into the vortex veins, yet some venous blood drains into the anterior episcleral vessels.

Characteristics of retinal and choroidal vessels

The differences between the retinal and choroidal circulation are summarized in Table 7.1.

Table 7.1 Characteristics of retinal and choroidal vessels

	Retinal vessels	Choroidal vessels
Anastomoses	None, i.e. end arteries	Interarterial shunts, between medium-sized arteries
Capillary size	Tubular	Sinusodal
Capillary type	Continuous	Fenestrated
Tight junctions	Present	Absent
Permeability to molecules	Minimal if any	High
Transport systems for essential substances	Present	Not required
Permeability to fluorescein	None	High
Permeability to indocyanin green (ICG)	None	Minimal

Clinical points

Fluorescein

Fluorescein is commonly used to study the retinal circulation. Normal retinal vessel does not leak fluorescein into the surrounding areas. However, in certain diseases, the abnormal retinal vessel would leak and can be picked up by fluorescein angiography (see Chapter 17 on fluorescein and its uses).

Indocyanin green

Indocyanin green is a new technique to study the choroidal circulation. As it is almost completely bound with protein, it does not easily pass through the vessel walls including choriocapillaris. It is useful in the identification of occult choriodal neovascularization. Clinical use is still very limited.

Ocular blood pressure and blood flow

Blood pressure in retinal and choroidal vessels

- Pressure in the retinal arteries is 25% below that of the ophthalmic artery.
- The pressure in the episcleral vessels is 7.2 mmHg below IOP.
- Uveal venous pressure is constant if IOP is between 10 and 15 mmHg.

- IOP >15 mmHg, the uveal venous pressure is directly proportional to IOP.
- This might be due to partial collapse of the intrascleral venous plexus.

Systemic blood pressure and ocular blood flow

- Uveal blood flow is proportional to arterial pressure.
- Oxygen saturation is constant despite reduced arterial pressure.
- Sudden changes of blood pressure do not change retinal vessel diameter.

Autoregulation

- Perfusion pressure of the retinal vessels is the difference between the mean arterial pressure and the IOP.
- Autoregulation in the retinal vessels allows constant blood flow over a wide range of perfusion pressures.
- The mechanism of autoregulation is unknown, but there are two major theories.
- Myogenic theory suggests that vasodilatation and vasoconstriction to maintain blood flow are effected by cell-to-cell transmission between adjacent smooth muscle cells from the periphery.
- Local metabolite theory proposes that metabolites are produced by retinal vessels experiencing local alterations in retinal blood flow.
- Autonomic nervous system regulates uveal circulation.

Intraocular pressure (IOP) and ocular blood flow

- As IOP increases, the velocity of retinal blood flow decreases, but overall blood flow remains constant until perfusion pressure is reduced by 63%.
- The constant retinal blood flow is maintained by vessels dilatation.
- In very high IOP, a rapid decrease in retinal blood flow occurs.
- Reactive increase of retinal blood flow occurs after sudden reduction of a persistently elevated IOP.

- Uveal blood flow also decreases with increased IOP.
- The arteriovenous oxygen differences increases with raised IOP.

Retinal blood flow and mean circulation time

- There is no precapillary sphincters in the retinal vessels.
- There are also no preferential channels for the blood to flow through.
- The retinal blood flow is about 2% of the total ocular blood flow.
- The average time taken for blood to flow from the retinal artery to vein is about 5 seconds.
- The estimated retinal blood flow is about 170 ml/100g/min.

Uveal blood flow

- The choroid captures about 65%, ciliary body 28% and the iris 5% of the total ocular blood flow.
- The total choroidal blood flow is about 0.5% of the total cardiac output.
- The relatively high blood flow to the choroid with minimal change in the arteriovenous oxygen difference indicates that the choroid attempt to maintain a high PO_2 in the retina to facilitate the dark current.

Oxygen saturation in ocular blood vessels

- Venous oxygen saturation is about 90% in the ciliary vein.
- The arteriovenous oxygen difference is about 0.9 ml/100 ml.
- Calculated oxygen consumption is about 0.7 ml/100 g/min.

Effects of inhaled gases upon ocular blood vessels

In breathing 100% oxygen

- The oxygen saturation in retinal veins increases by 50%.
- The retinal arteries decrease in diameter by 12% and retinal venous diameter by 15%.

- However, choroidal blood flow is virtually unchanged.
- The vasoconstriction effect in retinal vessels can cause irreversible damage to premature babies (retinopathy of prematurity).

In breathing 10% carbon dioxide with air

- Vasodilatation of retinal vessels.
- Increase of choroidal blood flow.

Chapter 8

Retina and neural pathways

Outline

The neurons of the retina are divided into three layers. The photoreceptors form the outer layer, whilst the bipolar cells, horizontal cells and amacrine cells in the intermediate layer with ganglion cells forming the inner layer. These neurons are supported by the glial cells called the Muller cells. The photoreceptors are intimately apposed to the retinal pigment epithelium which is apposed to Bruch's and the choroid. The ganglion cell axons converge to exit the eye as the optic nerve (see Figure 8.1).

Retina and neural pathways   61

The nasal half of the optic nerve fibres cross in the optic chiasma and synapse in the lateral geniculate nucleus on the contralateral side. The optic radiation relays the visual information to the visual cortex in the occipital lobes.

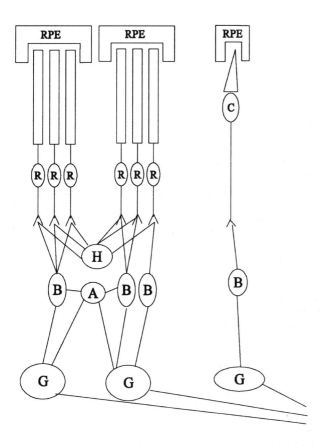

Figure 8.1 Diagrammatic illustration of the retina. Althouth horizontal cells and amacrine cells are not shown in the cones system, they are also present similar to that shown in the rods system. RPE = retinal pigment epithelium, R = rods, C = cones, H = horizontal cells, B = bipolar cells, A = amacrine cells, G = ganglion cells

Retinal pigment epithelium

The retinal pigment epithelium (RPE) is a single layer of epithelial cells between the Bruch's membrane and the neurosensory retina. Its proximity to the choroid allows the access of nutrients and deposition of metabolites for the neurosensory retina. Yet the tight junctions between the RPE cells form the outer blood–retina barrier which stops the free movement of large molecules and cells to the neurosensory retina.

The RPE cells recycle the visual pigment and phagocytose outer segment discs of photoreceptors. There is some evidence that their failure might be a cause of age-related macular degeneration. The latter is the leading cause of blindness in the Western world.

The RPE cells contain large amounts of melanin. This allows the absorption of light and reduces scattering so that a clear retinal image can be formed. The melanin also absorbs the thermal laser energy and forms the basis of ophthalmic laser therapy.

Main functions of the retinal pigment epithelium

- Providing nutrients for the photoreceptors.
- Active transportation of metabolites, lipids and ions.
- Outer blood–retina barrier.
- Regeneration and storage of visual pigment.
- Phagocytose outer segment discs of photoreceptors.
- Absorption of light by the melanin.

Photoreceptors

Differences between rods and cones

There are two main types of photoreceptors, namely rods and cones. Their function and histological morphology are distinctly different. They lie on the outermost layer of the neurosensory retina adjacent to the retinal pigment epithelium. The rods are responsible for night vision and the cones for colour and daytime vision. The latter are concentrated in the fovea and provide high visual resolution. Their differences are summarized in Table 8.1.

Table 8.1 Differences between rods and cones

	Rods	Cones
Numbers	120 million per eye	7 million per eye
Distribution	Uniformly distributed throughout the eye except fovea	Red and green sensitive cones concentrated in fovea, blue sensitive comes near fovea. Less concentrated elsewhere.
Sensitivity to light	High sensitivity	Lower sensitivity
Outer segments	Closed discs	Open discs
Photopigment	More, in membranous discs inside the outer segment	Less, incorporated in folds of the outer segment membrane
Function	Night vision	Daytime and colour vision
Connections	Many rods link to each retinal ganglion cell	One cone to one ganglion cell in fovea
Receptive fields	Larger	Smaller and hence better acuity
Directional sensitivity	Sensitive to light rays with wide angle of incidence	More specific directional sensitivity

Photochemistry in the photoreceptors

The visual cycle begins with the photoisomerization of the 11-*cis* retinal bound to opsin (photopigments) to the all-*trans* isomer. After the generation of the electrophysiologic signals, the photopigments are regenerated in the RPE.

Photopigments

Photopigments consist of the 11-*cis* retinal combined with an opsin. They are presented in the outer segments of photoreceptors.

There are four forms of opsin:

- rhodopsin   rods (maximum absorption 507 nm)
- erythrolabe   red sensitive cones (570 nm)
- chlorolabe   green sensitive cones (535 nm)
- cyanolabe   blue sensitive cones (440 nm)

Bleaching and regeneration of photopigments

The word 'bleaching' was first used by the nineteenth century physiologists to describe the change in colour of isolated retina after exposure to light. It is now generally used to described the physiological process of photoisomerization of photopigments (11-*cis* retinal + opsin) into all-*trans* retinal and free opsin (see Figure 8.2).

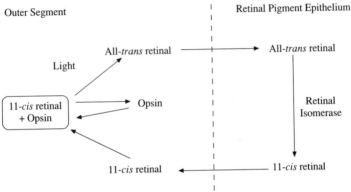

Figure 8.2 Bleaching and regeneration of photopigments

- Photon (light) enters outer segment.
- Absorbed by photopigment.
- Isomerization from 11-*cis* to all-*trans* retinal by light.
- Separation of retinal from opsin.
- Receptor membrane potential is generated (*vide infra*).
- All-*trans* retinal is transported to pigment epithelium.
- Regenerates into 11-*cis* isomer in the pigment epithelium.
- Returns to the outer segment and binds with opsin.

Photoreceptor cell renewal

Continuous synthesis of outer segment discs at the base of the outer segment is coupled with the continuous phagocytosis and degradation of shed discs by the RPE cells. Light plays an important role in the disc shedding process.

- Rods   Shed in the presence of light
- Cones   Shed in the dark

Phototransduction

The photoreceptor is unique in that a steady current flows along its plasma membrane in the absence of stimulation (called dark current). In the dark, the inner retina is electrically positive compared with the tips of the outer segments of photoreceptors. The current is generated by the Na/K 'pump' in the inner segment which actively removes sodium from the cell. The sodium enters the cell passively through the sodium channels in the plasma membrane of the outer segment.

Light induces photoisomerization of photopigments that closes these sodium channels in the outer segment. The intracellular sodium is markedly reduced and the plasma membrane potential changes from –40 mV to –75 mV. This hyperpolarization is transmitted to the synapse at the inner end of the photoreceptor and communicated with other retinal cells (see Figure 8.3).

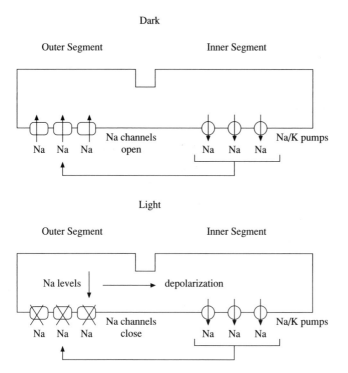

Figure 8.3 Phototransduction

For many years, it was uncertain how the sodium channels are closed by the release of opsin from photoisomerization. In addition, the system is very sensitive, and the absorption of a single photon of light by a single molecule of opsin reduces conductance through the plasma membrane by about 3%.

Membranous discs in the outer segments

It was found that there were other proteins present in the membranous discs in the outer segments of photoreceptors. The major proteins were as follows:

- cGMP phosphodiesterase.
- Transducin.
- Photopigments.

Light-triggered cGMP cascade

The sensitivity of the system is increased by the light-induced cGMP cascade.

- Light isomerizes 11-*cis* retinal to all-*trans* retinal.
- The isomerized molecules diffuse in the membrane.
- It activates a number of molecules of transducin.
- This catalyses the reaction of converting GDP into GTP.
- GTP binding can liberate α-GTP subunits (500 by each rhodopsin).
- α- GTP subunits disinhibits cGMP phosphodiesterase.
- Rapid hydrolysis of cGMP occurs (500 by each phosphodiesterase).
- Closes the outer segment sodium channels.

Other retinal cells

Photoreceptor potential is transmitted to the ganglion cells through two pathways. It can be connected directly through the bipolar cells. The signals can also be transferred indirectly through horizontal cells, bipolar cells and amacrine cells before reaching the ganglion cells (see Figure 8.1).

Horizontal cells

- Contact a wide area of photoreceptors.
- Electrically coupled to one another via gap junctions.
- Each photoreceptor is in contact with at least one horizontal cell.

Amacrine cells

- Many different types.
- Link bipolar and ganglion cells.
- Involved in complex circuits giving ganglion cells different field properties.

Bipolar cells

- Have circular receptive fields.
- Detect difference in luminance between an inner circle and a surrounding annulus.
- Excited by light in the centre of their receptive field — ON bipolar cells.
- Excited by dark in the centre of their receptive field — OFF bipolar cells.
- They are linked to the corresponding ON and OFF-centre ganglion cells.

Ganglion cells

- Main output cells of the retina.
- The first action potential occurs in this layer.
- Respond to a variety of different properties of stimulus.
- The fibres form the optic nerve.
- Project to superior colliculus and lateral geniculate nucleus (LGN).

Classification of the ganglion cells

Group A (Y-cells)

- Relatively large.

- Wide dendritic fields.
- Fast-conducting myelinated axons in the optic nerve.
- Respond to low spatial frequencies.
- Have high contrast sensitivity.
- Very sensitive to movements.
- No response to colour contrasts.
- Project to the magnocellular layers of the LGN.

Group B (X-cells)

- Smaller and with smaller dendritic fields.
- Slower-conducting myelinated axons.
- Respond to high spatial frequencies.
- Poor contrast sensitivity.
- Show colour opponency.
- Project to the parvocellular layers of the LGN.

Group C (W-cells)

- Small cells.
- Non-myelinated fibre in optic nerve.
- Uncertain properties — might be responsible for pupillary and ocular reflexes.
- Project to a variety of nuclei.

Lateral geniculate nucleus (LGN)

- Six layers in total.
- Two (1 and 2) ventral magnocellular layers — group A ganglion cells.
- Four (3–6) dorsal paravocellular layers — group B ganglion cells.
- Layers 2, 3 and 5 receive input from ipsilateral eye.
- Layers 1, 4 and 6 from the contralateral eye.
- The differences between the magnocellular and paravocellular layers are summarized in Table 8.2.

Table 8.2 Differences in magnocellular and paravocellular layers

	Magnocellular layer	Paravocellular layer
Input	Group A ganglion cells	Group B ganglion cells
Function	Movement, texture and stereoscopic vision	Colour, spatial resolution, orientation selectivity and end-stopping (shape)
Projection	Layer 4Cα of primary visual cortex	Layer 4Cβ of primary visual cortex

Cerebral cortex involved in vision

Primary visual cortex (V1)

- Located in the occipital cortex on the walls of calcarine fissure.
- Inputs from LGN.
- Entire contralateral visual field is represented.

Other visual areas (V2–5)

- Located in the peristriate and more anterior cortex.
- Each area responsible for a specific aspect of visual perception.
- V2 — Stereopsis, colour and high acuity vision.
- V3 — Form perception.
- V4 — Colour vision.
- V5 — Movement.

Columnar organization of the visual cortex

The visual cortex is a complex structure. Many terms have been used by various authors to describe certain features of the columnar organization. Some of these terms will be briefly discussed here. Further details can be obtained from neuro-physiology textbooks.

Ocular dominance columns

- Temporal fields are projected on the contralateral hemisphere.
- Corresponding regions of each retina project to closely adjacent neurons in appropriate regions of V1.

- These neurons are arranged in ocular dominance columns.
- They are cells in one column which respond preferentially to inputs from one eye.
- Columns are arranged in short lines or stripes approximately 400–500 µm wide.
- Each individual and each hemisphere has a different pattern of these stripes.
- It is believed that these stripes form dynamically during early childhood development rather than being genetically determined. This forms the basis of current concepts in ambylopia (see Chapter 11 on binocular vision and ambylopia).

Orientation columns

- Neurons that share the same orientation preference are also arranged in columns.
- They lie in the interblob regions.
- Ocular dominance and orientation columns are, however, not congruent.

Cytochrome oxidase blobs

- Cells in the blobs also form columns.
- Their main function is in colour processing.
- Both blob and interblob cells form part of the ocular dominance stripes.

Hypercolumns

- This orderly arrangement of columns allow a small region of cortex to receive inputs from all possible receptive fields within a small region of visual space.
- This region is called a hypercolumn.
- An adjacent part of retina is represented in adjacent hypercolumns.
- Thus the whole visual field is analysed in an orderly topographic fashion.

Section B
Neurophysiology related to eye

Chapter 9

Pupil and accommodation

The testing of pupillary reaction forms part of the clinical ophthalmic examination. It is useful to identify the location of the pathology. Normal pupils would constrict with light and accommodation (focus on a near object). The former is a brain stem reflex with no cerebral involvement whilst the latter involves the cerebral cortex.

Anatomical consideration of pupillary responses

Light reflexes

- Retinal ganglion cells axon leave the eye via the optic nerve.
- About half of the fibres decussate to the contralateral optic tract in the optic chiasm.

- Approximately two-thirds of the way along the optic tract, some of the axons enter the superior coliculus and synapse in the pretectal nucleus.
- The signal is then passed to the Edinger–Westphal (oculomotor) nuclei on both sides via intercalated neurons.
- The parasympathetic outflow travels with the inferior division of third cranial nerve (oculomotor) into the eye via the ciliary ganglion.
- The iris sphincter muscle responses to the signals and constricts the pupils.
- As the signal is passed to both nuclei, light information given to one eye is passed on to both pupils equally.
- The constriction of the ipsilateral pupil to the stimulus is called the direct light reflex.
- The constriction of the contralateral pupil is called the consensual light reflex.

Pupillary near response

- Upon focus on a near object, the eyes converge, the lenses accommodate and the pupils constrict; these form the near synkinesis triad.
- It is believed that the peristriate cortex (area 19) at the upper end of the calcarine fissure in the occipital cortex is the origin of the near synkinesis.
- The neurological pathway is more ventrally located than the pretectal afferent limb of the light reflexes upon the Edinger–Westphal (oculomotor) nucleus.
- The final pathway via the oculomotor nerve and ciliary ganglion is identical to the light reflexes.

Dilator muscle of the iris

- This muscle is innervated by sympathetic fibres.
- The neuron originates in posterior hypothalamus and tracts through the brain stem to the C8–T2 level of the spinal cord.
- Pre-ganglionic neurons leave the cord and terminate in the superior cervical ganglion at the base of the skull.
- Post-ganglionic neurons ascend with the internal carotid artery joining the ophthalmic nerve in the cavernous sinus.

- It then enters the orbit through the superior orbital fissure and enter the eye via the long ciliary nerve.

Pathophysiology of abnormal pupillary responses

Relative afferent pupillary defect (Marcus Gunn pupil)

- When the afferent pathway (retina to optic chiasm) of one eye is damaged, a light stimulus to the affected eye will not be able to induce a pupillary reflex.
- Nevertheless, the light stimulus to the normal eye would induce the normal direct and consensual pupillary reflexes.
- By swinging a light from the normal eye (constriction by normal light reflexes) to the abnormal eye (no constriction), the pupils would dilate and vice versa.
- As dilatation is easier to see than constriction, the former is used clinically.
- Bearing in mind that the defect might not always be complete, the dilatation could be quite subtle; in this situation a bright light in a semi-darkened room would maximize the change in pupil sizes.

Light — near dissociation

- This term is used to describe patients with abnormal light reflexes but a normal near response.
- The classical example is the Argyll Robertson pupils associated with neurosyphilis.
- It is believed the lesion is in the Sylvian aqueduct in the brain stem interfering the light reflex fibres; the more ventrally located near response fibres are spared.
- There is no known condition that affects near response only, hence if the light reflexes are normal, the examination of the near pupillary response is unnecessary.

Adie's pupil

- This is an idiopathic condition which mostly affects young women and tends to be bilateral.
- Dilated pupil with poor or no light reflexes.

- Slow constriction occurs with prolonged near effort and redilatation is also slow. Accommodation paresis is common initially but tends to recover.
- Sectorial denervation of the iris sphincter is present.
- Majority demonstrates cholinergic supersensitivity to weak pilocarpine (0.1%) solutions which forms the basis of the clinical test.
- The lesion is believed to be in the ciliary ganglion or the short posterior ciliary nerves.
- Aberration regeneration is mainly (97%) to the ciliary muscle, hence the recovery of the accommodation.
- When it is associated with the absence of deep tendon reflexes, it is called the Holmes–Adie syndrome.

Horner's syndrome

- The affected side shows miosis of the pupil, mild ptosis (drooping lid), anhydrosis of face (reduce sweating) and apparent enophthalmos.
- Cocaine blocks the noradrenaline receptors at the myoneural junction and hence prolongs the action of noradrenaline upon the dilator muscle.
- The normal pupil will dilate but not the affected pupil, as there is no noradrenaline present in the first place and hence no prolonging effect. Horner's syndrome is thus confirmed.
- Hydroxyamphetamine causes release of noradrenaline from the nerve endings at the myoneural junction, thereby stimulating the dilator muscle.
- The post-ganglionic neuron has to be intact in order to have noradrenaline at the nerve ends.
- Subnormal dilatation with hydroxyamphetamine therefore implies a post-ganglionic lesion.
- Thus, the cocaine test confirms the diagnosis and hydroxyamphetamine test identifies lesion in the post-ganglionic neuron.
- Anhydrosis of the affected side of the face only occurs if the lesion involves the sympathetic pathway proximal to the bifurcation of the common carotid artery, since the sudomotor fibres travel with the external carotid.

Hutchison pupil of the comatose

- Unilateral dilated and poorly reactive pupil in comatose patient.
- Due to ipsilateral expanding intracranial supratentorial mass such as a subdural haematoma.
- It causes downward displacement of the hippocampal gyrus and uncal herniation across the tentorial edge with entrapment of the third cranial nerve.
- The pupillomotor fibres travel in the peripheral portion of the third nerve and are subject to early damage from compression.
- Further herniation can lead to compression of the brain stem followed by respiratory arrest, and this situation needs urgent neurosurgical intervention.

Pupil during sleep

- In sleeping, the cortical inhibitory input to the Edinger–Westphal nucleus is reduced and hence the pupils are small but reactive to light.
- On opening the eyelid of a person who pretends to be sleeping, the pupil is initially dilated (because the light is blocked by the closing lid) and constricts rapidly when the lid is opened.

Accommodation

The normal eye focuses images of distant objects on the retina at rest, for the eye to focus a near object, an increase of ocular refractive power is required. This is called accommodation.

Mechanism of accommodation

- As mentioned, the near synkinesis involves convergence of both eyes, miosis and the accommodation of the lenses.
- It is probably originated from the peristriate cortex (area 19) at the upper end of the calcarine fissure in the occipital cortex.
- When the ciliary muscle is relaxed, the tension on the zonules allow the young lens to mould by the capsule into a flattened form.

- Contraction of the ciliary muscle causes relaxation of the zonules and the tension on the capsule is relieved, the lens attains a more spherical shape.
- This results in an increase in the dioptric power of the lens and allows a near object to come into focus.

Changes in lens shape during accommodation

- The principal change in the lens is seen at the anterior surface.
- The anterior surface bulges centrally.
- The peripheral anterior surface and the posterior lens surface have only minimal change in curvature.

Stimulus for accommodation

- The mechanism is not completely understood.
- Apparent size and distance of an object, blur, chromatic aberration, oscillation of accommodation and scanning movements are all believed to have a role in the controlling mechanism.

Presbyopia

- This is defined as the normal progressive reduction on the amplitude of accommodation with age.
- The amplitude of accommodation is the amount that the eye can alter its refractive power in focusing on a far object and a near object.
- At the age of 10, the amplitude of accommodation is about 14 dioptres, reducing to about 2 dioptres at the age of 50 and less than 1 dioptre in the over-60s.
- This is the reason that older people need reading glasses to help them accommodate in order to read.
- The reduction in capsule elasticity in the senile lens has a role in causing presbyopia.
- The progressive hardening of the lens, probably secondary to the alteration in the structural protein of the lens and the increase in adhesion between lens fibre, also contributes to the loss of the amplitude of accommodation.

AC/A ratio (accommodative convergence/accommodation)

- This is defined as the accommodative convergence exerted in response to one unit of accommodation, it is normally about 3–5 to 1.

- In other words, 1 dioptre of accommodation would normally induce 3–5 dioptres of accommodative convergence.

- It is measured by performing prism cover test at 6 metres and at 33 cm, the change of the accommodative convergence divides by 3 (the accommodative power requires to focus at 33 cm) gives the AC/A ratio.

- Abnormal AC/A ratios are seen in certain patients with strabismus.

Chapter 10

Ocular movement

Outline

Type of ocular movements
    Ductions
    Versions
        Secondary positions of gaze
        Tertiary positions of gaze
        Cycloversion
        Positions of gaze
        Yoke muscle
    Vergences
        AC/A ratio (accommodative convergence/accommodation)
        Fusional vergences

Action of the extraocular muscles
    Sherrington's law of reciprocal innervation
    Hering's law
Supranuclear control of ocular movements
    Saccade
    Pursuit
    Vestibular
    Vergence
    Paramedian pontine reticular formation
Nystagmus

In the description of ocular movements, terminology can be confusing. It is worthwhile to understand them, so that the orthoptist report becomes more meaningful.

Type of ocular movements

Eye movements are of three types; ductions, versions and vergences

Ductions

- Monocular eye movements.
- Consist of adduction, abduction, elevation, depression, intorsion and extorsion.
- Adduction means the eye turns nasally.
- Abduction means the eye turns temporally.
- Elevation means the eye looks up.
- Depression means the eye looks down.
- Intortion means the upper pole of the eye rotates nasally.
- Extortion means the upper pole of the eye rotates temporally.
- Agonist — primary muscle moving the eye in any given direction, e.g. medial rectus on adduction.
- Synergist — muscle acts in conjunction with the agonist, e.g. superior and inferior recti on adduction.
- Antagonist — muscle acts in the opposite direction to the agonist, e.g. lateral rectus on adduction.

Versions

- Binocular eye movements.
- Both eyes move symmetrically and synchronously in the same direction.

Secondary positions of gaze

- Dextroversion   right gaze
- Laevoversion   left gaze
- Elevation   up gaze
- Depression   down gaze

Tertiary positions of gaze

- Dextroelevation   up and right
- Dextrodepression   down and right
- Laevoelevation   up and left
- Laevodepression   down and left

Cycloversion

- Dextrocycloversion   rotation of both eyes to the right
- Laevocycloversion   rotation of both eyes to the left

Positions of gaze

- There are nine positions of gaze which are the primary position with the four secondary and four tertiary positions of gaze (*vide supra*).
- However, only six of these are called cardinal positions of gaze, which fits into the concept of the yoke muscle (*vide infra*).
- These are dextroversion, laevoversion, dextroelevation, laevo-elevation, dextrodepression and laevodepression.

Yoke muscle

- A muscle on one eye is paired with a muscle on the other eye in a cardinal position of gaze.
- For example, in laevoversion, the two yoke muscles are the left lateral rectus and right medial rectus.

Vergences

- Binocular movement.
- Both eyes move symmetrically and synchronously in opposite directions.
- Convergence — both eyes turn inwards.
- Divergence — both eyes turn outwards.

AC/A ratio (accommodative convergence/accommodation)

- This ratio is the amount of convergence measured in prism dioptres per unit change in accommodation.
- The normal value is between 3 and 5 prism dioptres.
- High ratio may cause convergent squint.

Fusional vergences

- The ability for the eyes to correct retinal image disparity.
- Controlled phoria (latent squint).
- Fusional amplitude refers to the maximal amount of eye movement produced by fusional vergences.
- Measured by prisms bar or synoptophore.

- Normal fusional convergence amplitude is about 15 prism dioptres for distance and 25 for near.
- The amplitude can be improved by orthoptic exercise to treat convergence insufficiency.

Action of the extraocular muscles

Six extraocular muscles control ocular movement. The details are summarized in Table 10.1.

Table 10.1 The extraocular muscles

	Medial rectus	Lateral rectus	Superior rectus	Inferior rectus	Superior oblique	Inferior oblique
Supplied by	CN III	CN VI	CN III (contralateral)	CN III	CN IV	CN III
Main Action	Adduction	Abduction	Elevation on abduction	Depression on abduction	Depression on adduction	Elevation on adduction
Secondar Action	None	None	Adduction and intorsion	Adduction and extorsion	Abduction and intorsion	Abduction and extorsion

Sherrington's law of reciprocal innervation

This law implies that increased innervation and contraction of a muscle is automatically associated with a reciprocal decrease in innervation and hence relaxation of its antagonist.

Hering's law

This law states that during any conjugate eye movement, equal and simultaneous innervation flows to the yoke muscles.

Supranuclear control of ocular movements

Saccade

- Fast voluntary eye movement.
- Velocity 300–700 degree/s.
- To bring images of interest onto the fovea.

- The correcting quick phase in nystagmus.
- Saccadic suppression: there is no sense of blurred image during saccades.
- Response to sudden peripheral visual, auditory or sensory stimulus.
- Generated by the frontal eye field (area 8 of the frontal lobe).
- The fronto–mesencephalic pathways pass through the internal capsule to decussate in the lower midbrain and terminate in the PPRF (paramedial pontine reticular formation) in the lower pons.
- PPRF is the horizontal gaze control centre.
- Stimulation of the left area 8 results in right gaze.

Pursuit

- Slow voluntary eye movement.
- Velocity 20–50 degree/s.
- To hold the image of a moving target on the fovea.
- Once the eyes have achieved macular fixation of a slowly moving target, the eyes will pursue at the velocity of the target in a smooth fashion.
- If the target is moving quicker than 50 degree/s, the eye will fall behind, saccadic movement will regain fixation and then the eye will pursue again, producing the characteristic cog-wheel pursuit eye movements.
- The parieto-occipito-temporal (POT) junction is believed to be the cortical centre for pursuit.
- The exact pathway is incompletely understood.
- It is observed to be an ipsilateral control.
- Right POT junction controls smooth pursuit to the right.

Vestibular

- Slow involuntary eye movement.
- Velocity 20–50 degree/s.
- To hold images on the retinal during brief head movements.
- The membranous labyrinth lies within the temporal bone, cushioned by perilymph.

- There are three semicircular canals and respective cristae, each in an ampulla, which sense head rotation.
- The utricle and saccule and their respective maculae sense head position.
- Stimulation of each set of semicircular canals precisely influences a particular pair of eye muscles.
- Information from the ampulla of the right horizontal semicircular canal is transmitted to the left PPRF, resulting in vestibular eye movement to the left.
- Information from the anterior and posterior semicircular canals results in combinations of rotary and vertical eye movements.

Vergence

- Slow eye movement.
- Velocity 20–50 degree/s.
- Carries the eyes in opposite directions.
- Near reflexes originate in area 19 and descend to the CN III nuclei, resulting in accommodation, miosis and convergence.

Paramedian pontine reticular formation (PPRF)

- This area serves as the starting point of the final common pathway for conjugate horizontal eye movements.
- It is often referred as the horizontal gaze centre.
- It is located in the mid-pons inferior to the medial longitudinal fasciculus (MLF).
- The major pathways are diagramatically illustrated in Figure 10.1 on page 86.

Nystagmus

- It is an involuntary to and fro eye movements.
- It can be described as jerk (fast and show phases present) or pendular (constant velocity).
- Physiological nystagmus — present in normal people, for example optokinetic nystagmus.
- Vestibular nystagmus — lesion in inner ear, usually jerk.

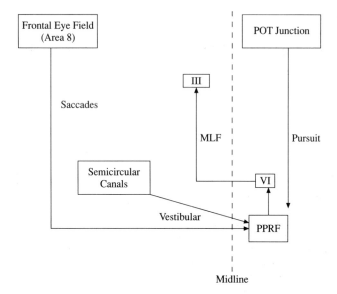

Figure 10.1 Diagrammatic representation of supranuclear horizontal eye movement control. III = Oculomotor nucleus; VI = Abducen nucleus; POT = Parieto-occipito-temporal; MLF = Medial longitudinal fasciculus; PPRF = Paramedian pontine reticular formation

- Gaze-evoked nystagmus — in brainstem lesion, usually jerk.
- Sensory nystagmus — secondary to poor vision in infancy, for example in congenital cataracts; usually pendular.
- Motor imbalance nystagmus — secondary to a specific lesion, for example see-saw nystagmus in chiasmal lesion or ataxic nystagmus in internuclear ophthalmoplegia.

Chapter 11

Binocular single vision and amblyopia

Outline

It is interesting to note that most animals have two eyes; this arrangement ensures a large visual field and enables the use of stereoscopic depth perception. The latter is commonly described as binocular single vision (BSV).

BSV involves complex neurophysiology concepts and many facets are not completely understood. The easiest way to consider BSV is to imagine that both eyes perceive a similar but slightly different image, by appreciating the disparity, a sense of depth is achieved.

In the investigation of BSV, there are some important basic concepts. They will be discussed in this chapter.

Corresponding retinal points and binocular disparity

- Imagine the retina of the two eyes as two sheets of graph papers with the fovea at the centre of each.
- A retinal point can be expressed by stating the horizontal and vertical distance from the fovea.
- A point so marked in one eye will have a corresponding point on the other eye, derived from the same data.
- These are called the corresponding retinal points.
- When a stimulus point falls on exactly the same retinal region (points) in both eyes, this is called zero binocular disparity.
- Hence, when a stimulus point falls on different retinal points in the eyes, the difference between the corresponding retinal point and the actual image point is called binocular disparity.
- A small binocular disparity can still be perceived as a single image; this range of fusion is called the Panum's area, and beyond that the patient will see double (diplopia).

Horopter

- When an observer fixates at infinity, there are a set of points in space having zero binocular disparity, i.e. in the same visual direction in space.
- The locus of these points is known as the horopter ('horizon of vision').
- The point horopter is a line in space passing through the point of fixation.
- In ophthalmology, fusion horopter is most commonly used; it is a three-dimensional volume in space that the locus of points in space appear binocularly fused to the observer.

Physiological basis of fusion and diplopia

It is well known that when a stimulus point falls on slightly different corresponding retinal points within the Panum's area, the observer can still manage to fuse the image to see a single image. When the disparity increases, two images will be seen. However, when the disparity is very large, one of the images will be suppressed and hence only one image is seen. The physiological basis of these phenomena is not fully understood; nevertheless, it is believed that there are four classes of neurons involved.

- Binocular corresponding — activated by exact corresponding points in both eyes.
- Binocular disparate — activated by disparity corresponding points.
- Monocular right — activated by stimulation of right eye.
- Monocular left — activated by stimulation of left eye.

Stimuli in the corresponding points

- When the stimuli are in corresponding points.
- Binocular corresponding — stimulated.
- Binocular disparate — not stimulated.
- Monocular right — stimulated.
- Monocular left — stimulated.

As all the three stimulated classes of neurons have the same visual direction, there is no conflict and the object of attention is hence seen as a single image.

Small disparity between stimuli

- When a small disparity is present.
- Binocular corresponding — not stimulated.
- Binocular disparate — stimulated.
- Monocular right — stimulated for a visual direction slightly to one side of the mean.
- Monocular left — stimulated for a visual direction slightly to the opposite side of the mean.

The two monocular visual directions are discriminably different if presented singly but they are integrated with the third set of responses from the binocular disparate class of neurons. This will give a fused image.

Large disparity between stimuli

- When there is a larger disparity.
- Binocular corresponding — not stimulated.
- Binocular disparate — not stimulated.
- Monocular right — stimulated in a different visual direction as compared with monocular left.
- Monocular left — stimulated in a different visual direction as compared with monocular right.

As the disparity increases, the binocular classes of neurons are no longer stimulated and hence no integration is possible; the two monocular classes have been stimulated in different visual directions and hence two images are seen (diplopia).

Very large disparity between stimuli

- When there is a very large disparity.
- Binocular corresponding — not stimulated.
- Binocular disparate — not stimulated.
- Monocular right — not stimulated.
- Monocular left — not stimulated.

It is believed that these classes of neurons are only stimulated when there is a small disparity. When there is a very large disparity, suppression occurs.

Binocular rivalry and suppression

- If two different images are projected to each eye within the same visual direction, the resulting conflict is resolved by temporal alternation between the two images.
- In other words, one image is seen at one time followed by seeing the other image.
- The suppression state is an inhibitory state.
- When there is a binocular mismatch, the higher stimulus strength in one eye causes a greater suppression on the other eye.
- Higher stimulus strength is defined in terms of luminance, contrast, movement or form sense.

Physiology of stereopsis

- As the eyes are horizontally separated in space, there is a slight disparate view of all objects located nearer than infinity.
- If both eyes fixate on an image which is moved closer to the observer, a difference in depth can be signaled by binocular disparity and convergence.
- The image shifts in a temporal direction in each eye, producing binocular disparity as the image falls on non-corresponding retinal points.
- At the same time, the eyes converge to the new vergence angle so as to reacquire bifoveal fixation; the difference in the vergence angle provides the cue to the new distance of the object.
- It is arguable that the change in vergence angle might be not as important as binocular disparity in view of the fact that some patients without BSV can converge well.

Development of binocular single vision

At birth, the retina and the optic pathways are not completely developed. Some degree of visual function is seen at about 6 weeks and fusion can be demonstrated as early as 6 months of age.

6 weeks

- First manifestation of fixation reflex.
- The eyes follow a light for a few degrees.
- Once fixation is interrupted, re-establishment is slow.

3 months

- Fixation in all fields of gaze.
- Re-establishes fixation instantly after interruption.

4–6 months

- Associate fixation with grasping movements.
- First clinical testing possible by using a base-out prism.
- To achieve fusion, the eye will converge (*vide infra*).

Worth's classification of binocular single vision

This classification is based on clinical examination using a synoptophore. A synoptophore is an instrument for the assessment of squint and BSV. It consists of two cylindrical tubes with a viewing eyepiece on one end. Pictures can be inserted in a slide carrier on the other end of each tube. The angle between the two tubes can be adjusted and the degree of the squint can be measured.

Simultaneous perception

- Simultaneous awareness of dissimilar but not antagonistic targets presented to each eye.
- One picture is smaller than the other so that the smaller picture is seen by the fovea and the other one is seen perifoveally.
- For example, a bird and a cage.

Fusion

- Blending of similar targets having only minor dissimilarity present to each eye.
- For example, a rabbit without a tail and a rabbit without the ears.
- The whole rabbit will be seen when fusion is present.
- The similar portions of each object (e.g. the body of the rabbit) incite a motor response called fusional vergence.
- The range of fusion can be tested by moving the arms of the synoptophore so that the eyes have to converge or diverge in order to maintain fusion.

Stereopsis

- Integrating of similar but disparate targets, obtaining a perception of stereopsis, i.e. a sense of depth.
- For example, two pictures of the same object which have been taken from slightly different angles.
- Nevertheless, some degree of depth perception can be achieved with monocular clues. In clinical testing, it is crucial to ensure the patient is not able to use these clues.

Amblyopia

Amblyopia has been defined as reduce visual acuity in the absence of organic dysfunction. In other words, the eye appears to be normal but the visual acuity is reduced despite refractive correction. This is commonly known as the 'lazy eye'.

In some patients, pathology can be found in the eye, but the visual acuity is worse than expected. This is also amblyopia. Furthermore, it is now known that amblyopia is associated with poor visual cortical development, hence organic dysfunction is present. Amblyopia is secondary to visual deprivation in the early part of life.

Uniocular visual deprivation in early childhood

- Induces competition between the cortical afferents.
- As a result of this competition, the cortical afferents tend to follow the visual pathway with visual (form sense) stimulation.
- Hence, there is a decrease in the size of lateral geniculate nucleus cells receiving input from affected eye.
- Morphological changes in the layer IV of visual cortex which receives the geniculate efferents are also apparent.

'Critical period'

- The term 'critical period' is used to describe the period of time that visual deprivation can cause amblyopia.
- In general, the longer the period of visual deprivation, the more likely it is to lead to severe amblyopia.
- However, the same length of visual deprivation at a different age leads to a different degree of amblyopia.
- The critical period is believed to begin at about 4 months and has maximum sensitivity at 6–9 months; it then declines until the age of 8.
- In other words, a short visual deprivation at the age of 6 months can cause profound amblyopia, whilst the same visual deprivation after the age of 8 will not cause amblyopia at all.
- This is very important in the management of amblyopia by patching (*vide infra*).

Clinical classification of amblyopia

Stimulus deprivation amblyopia

Optical media opacities, such as cataract or ptosis, cause visual deprivation and hence amblyopia. These opacities should be removed as soon as possible. However, in congenital cataract, it may prove difficult, as unilateral aphakia is a strong amblyogenic factor.

Anisometropic amblyopia

Anisometropia is present if the refractive errors of the two eyes are significantly different. The more ametropic eye has a constant blurred image on the fovea which leads to amblyopia.

Strabismic amblyopia

The image from the squinting eye is suppressed. This constant suppression leads to amblyopia. It can coexist with aniso-metropic amblyopia, and in fact, the latter might be the cause of the squint itself.

Management of amblyopia

- Removal of the amblyogenic agents, such as ptosis correction and refractive correction.
- Patch the good eye, so as the amblyopic eye has a competitive advantage.
- If patching is not possible due to poor compliance, atropine can be used to blur the image on the good eye; however, this treatment is only used as a last resort.
- It is important to bear in mind that extensive patching or atropinization can cause amblyopia in the good eye, although fortunately reversal is usually fast.

Chapter 12

Colour vision

   The electromagnetic spectrum extends from the cosmic rays and X-rays with very short wavelength to radio waves used in broadcasting with very long wavelength. Visible light is a narrow part of this spectrum with wavelengths between about 400 nm and 700 nm. Different wavelengths of light are perceived as different colours by the human eye.

History of the development in colour vision theory

- Isaac Newton spread the light spectrum of white sunlight using a prism in 1666.

- He speculated that light sets up vibrations in the optic nerves that are tuned to respond to each colour.

- In 1802, Thomas Young suggested it is impossible to have receptors for each colour in a particular point of the retina.

- He postulated the Principle theory of three principle colours.

- Helmholtz elaborated Young's theory in 1863, that each receptor responds maximally to a particular region of the spectrum, but they all respond to other parts of the spectrum in a lesser extent.
- Hering proposed three kinds of 'catching material', two substances providing signals about colour and one for blackness or whiteness.
- The three substances were responsible for producing warm (white, yellow, red) and cold (black, blue, green) colours. Hering suggested that each warm colour is paired with a cold colour in each substance.
- It is now known that there are three types of cone receptors, as Young and Helmholtz suggested. The subsequent neural pathways that compare the outputs of the different receptor types (spectrally opponent interactions) is similar to that suggested by Hering.

Types of cones

- Blue cones: peak spectral sensitivities at 440–450 nm.
- Green cones: peak spectral sensitivities at 535–555 nm.
- Red cones: peak spectral sensitivities at 570–590 nm.

Neuronal control of colour vision

- The exact role in colour processing of different cells in the neural pathway is far from clear.
- The horizontal cells show two types of response, the luminosity response appears to signal brightness and the chromatic response that is hyperpolarizing for one colour spectrum (say red–green) and depolarizing for another colour (blue–yellow).
- The bipolar cells seem to carry colour coded receptive fields; for example red light strikes in the centre of these fields caused hyperpolarization and green light in the surroundings caused depolarization.
- The role of amacrine cells is unknown; it is believed they take the role of 'automatic colour control' to allow the normal eye to experience colour constancy, in the way that a white object continues to be perceived as white even though the spectral composition of the light falling on it, is markedly altered.

- Colour coded receptive fields are present in the ganglion cells, which are excited by red light in the centre of the receptive field and inhibited by green light in the periphery.
- There is also evidence of double opponency in which maximum firing occurs in both a red centre surrounded by a green ring or a green centre surrounded by a red ring.
- In the lateral geniculate nucleus, there are four types of spectrally opponent cells, two with red and green antagonism (+R/-G and +G/-R) and two with blue and yellow antagonism (+B/-Y) and (+Y/-B).
- The red–green cells seem clearly to have input from just the red and green cones, but the input of the blue–yellow cells is less certain. It is, however, believed that the blue cones provide the blue arm of the input whilst the combination of the red and green cones provides the yellow arm of the input.
- In the visual cortex, colour specific cells are present. They appear to respond briskly to monochromatic light but show no response to white light at all.
- The presence of double opponent cells has also been demonstrated.
- The colour specific cortical cells seem to be most numerous in the post-striate region of the cortex just anterior to the classic visual areas.

Colour description

The description of colour is very subjective; what one individual sees as faded red, another might describe as pink. Precise identification of colour is important in items such as textiles, paint, food and so on. There are two commonly used systems.

The Commission International de l'Eclairage (CIE) system

- It was well known, even as far back as the time of Newton, that any colours can be made by a careful mixture of three primary colours, namely red, green and blue.
- For practical reasons, the CIE chose to use unreal primaries called X, Y and Z.
- In this system, all negative values in representing colours are excluded.

- The relative amounts of each of the X, Y and Z primaries in a mixture required to match that colour are expressed as chromaticity co-ordinates (x, y, z).
- As the co-ordinates represent relative amounts of primary, only two of them are required to specify the chromaticity of a colour.
- The luminance quality (brightness) of a colour is expressed separately as the Y value which is the amount of the Y primary.

Munsell colour system

- Another method uses to describe a colour is by identifying three subjective attributes, the hue, value and chroma.
- All colours in the Munsell system are represented in a cylinder, similar to a round card filing system.
- The hue dimension is located on the circumference of the cylinder, it contains ten basic colours which are subdivided into ten equal steps, giving an array of 100 hues around the circle.
- The value dimension is indicated by moving up or down the cylinder for a given hue; the lightest expression of that colour is at the top and the darkest at the bottom.
- The chroma (whiteness) dimension is the degree of saturation of the colour and expresses as the distance from the axis of the cylinder; colours aligned vertically all have the same chroma; at the axis, the colour is so desaturated that it will look white or grey to the eye, whilst as far away from the axis, the colour becomes more saturated and looks more vivid.

Anomalies of colour vision

- Truly colour-blind individuals are few.
- Colour defective vision is present in about 10% of all males and 1% of females as a X-linked recessive condition.
- Red–green defectives may be trichromatic with two normal and one abnormal cones, referred to as deuteranomalous (green) and protanomalous (red).
- They can also be dichromatic with one missing photopigment, referred to as deuteranopes (green) and protanopes (red).

- Hereditary colour defects involving the blue cone are rare, and are termed tritan defects.

- Acquired colour defect occurs in a number of ocular and systemic diseases, and can affect both the red–green and blue–yellow axis.

- In general, ganglion cells and optic nerve diseases tend to affect the red–green axis whilst inner retinal diseases affect the blue–yellow axis. Few exceptions have been reported, for instance, glaucoma, a ganglion cell disease, is associated with blue–yellow axis defect rather than the red–green axis.

Clinical colour testing

Pseudoisochromatic plates

- These plates are made up of coloured dots.

- The coloured dots are arranged in such a fashion that the normal eye can group certain colours together to produce a figure which is usually a letter or a number.

- The dots of the figures and background cover a wide range of lightness values so that the recognition of the figures can be made only by colour discrimination of either hue or saturation.

- The Ishihara colour plate is the most commonly used pseudoisochromatic plate.

Farnsworth Munsell 100 hue test

- Despite its name, the 100 hue test consists of only 85 coloured plastic tops selected from the hue circle.

- The 85 different coloured caps are selected to represent equal steps of colour difference around a complete colour circle.

- The caps are divided into four groups, each representing a quadrant of the colour circle.

- As the saturation and luminance is equal, this is a hue discrimination test.

- The subject is given one tray at a time and allowed 2 minutes with each tray to arrange the colours in serial order of their hue.

- Colour defectives are found to produce their errors in characteristic sections of the colour circle.

- The total number of errors allows a measure of severity.
- It is, however, a time-consuming test (takes about 15–20 minutes).

Farnsworth D-15 test

- Instead of using 85 caps, 15 caps are used to form a colour circle.
- All 15 caps are presented to the patient at the same time, hence the patient can confuse colours across the different quadrants of the colour circle.
- Again, there is characteristic pattern of red–green and blue–yellow defects.
- It is a good screening test and takes much less time to perform.

Chapter 13

Higher visual processing

Visual processing is a complex neurophysiological process. Despite extensive research in this field, there are still many uncertain areas. It is believed that there are different types of neurons response to different type of stimulus. Some of them are stimulated by contrast illuminations, others by change of contours.

Visual phenomena such as dark and light adaptation, after images and critical fusion frequency will be briefly discussed in this chapter.

Centre–surround receptive fields

- Many cells have action potentials, even in the dark.
- Light or dark spots may increase or decrease the frequency of action potentials.
- Excitatory and inhibitory regions are arranged in the form of an annulus surrounding a central circle.
- In an ON centre unit, light stimulates the centre but inhibits the surrounding areas.

- In an OFF centre unit, the opposite occurs.
- Hence, uniform stimulation throughout the field gives no or little response.
- Receptive fields respond to contrast in illumination.
- Similar colour sensitive units are also present (see Chapter 12 Colour vision).
- These receptive fields are present in ganglion cells and geniculate cells.

Orientation sensitivity

- Many cells respond to contours.
- Simple cells respond to bars or edges with a particular orientation in a fixed visual space.
- Complex cells respond to bars or edges with particular orientation and optimal width but placed anywhere in a larger visual space.
- Hypercomplex cells respond to bars or edges end or change direction within their receptive field.
- Periodic pattern sensitive cells respond to specific pattern with a small range of variation in their spatial frequency, e.g. gratings.

High acuity vision

- Acuity is not limited by optics, but by the resolving power of the retina.
- In the fovea, the limit is set by the distance between two cones (2.5 μm) and the packed cell density.
- Away from the fovea, the receptive fields get larger and acuity lower as the distance between adjacent cones also increases.

Dark adaptation

The sensitivity of the eye depends on the ambient light intensity. There is a gradual increase in sensitivity to dimmer light when going into a darker environment. This phenomenon is called dark adaptation.

Mechanisms of dark adaptation

- Pupil dilatation.
- Neural changes medicated by amacrine cells in retina.
- Increase in receptor sensitivity (most important).

Biphasic curve of dark adaptation

- Regeneration of photopigments from their bleached form.
- Cones take 10 min.
- Rods take 30 min — as they contain more photopigment and hence take longer (see Figure 13.1).

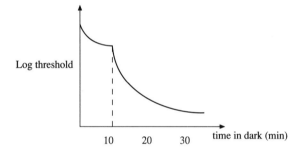

Figure 13.1 Biphasic curve of dark adaptation, vertical line = rod/cone break

Light adaptation

Similarly, light adaptation occurs. It is, however, much faster and takes about 3–5 minutes by the following mechanisms:

- Pupil constriction.
- Bleaching of photopigments.

Maximum sensitivity of the eye

- Scotopic (dark adapted)   507 nm (green)
- Photopic (light adapted)   555 nm (yellow)

The shift of maximum sensitivity from scotopic to photopic conditions is known as Purkinje shift.

After-images

- Visual sensations outlast the stimulus.
- A negative after-image is visualized as a reversed of the original stimulus, that is light areas are dark and vice versa. It is seen commonly by staring at a bright image for a few moments and then transferring the gaze to a dimly illuminated even background.
- A positive after-image is visualized as the original stimulus. It is seen commonly by staring at a dark pattern in very bright light for a few seconds, after which the eyes are occluded.
- It is believed that intense stimulation causes a lasting change in the level of bleached photopigment which causes this phenomena. There is also some evidence that it is partly of central origin.

Critical fusion frequency (CFF)

- Flickering stimulus appears to be continuous.
- Depends on the frequency of action potentials fired by ganglion cells.
- In dim light, could be less than 10 Hz (cycles/s).
- In bright light, around 60 Hz.
- This phenomena allows us to watch movies as continuous moving pictures.

Section C
Associated disciplines

Chapter 14

Immunology and the eye

Outline

The immune system allows us to fight against foreign materials such as micro-organisms. In some occasions, however, it can become an enemy. Hypersensitivity of the immune system can cause more damage than the foreign insult. It is also the source for a whole range of auto-immune diseases which can affect the eye in many ways. In transplantation surgery, such as corneal transplant, the immune response plays an important role for graft rejection leading to graft failure.

The immune system

All cells in the immune system are developed from the bone marrow stem cells. The lymphoid lineage produces T-lymphocytes and B-lymphocytes, whilst the myeloid pathway gives rise to monocytes and polymorphs. They are all white blood cells. Polymorphs are subdivided into neutrophils, eosinophils and basophils whilst the monocytes can be transformed into tissue macrophages.

In response to a foreign body, the immune system induces an acute inflammatory response which is non-specific and an immune response which is specific to the foreign material.

Acute inflammation

- This is a non-specific response to range of insults.
- Infection, trauma, radiation and chemical injury can cause the response.
- The insult activates the Hageman factor in plasma which in turn stimulates a range of cascade systems.
- The cascade systems lead to the release of various substances.
- Two recognizable stages, the vascular and cellular phase.
- The acute response lasts for 24–48 hours.
- Unlike the immune response, there is no 'memory', that is it responds to the same insult in a similar fashion.

Vascular phase

- Vasodilatation is mediated by histamine, kinins and prostaglandins.
- Histamine is released from mast cells; it increases vascular permeability and causes vasodilatation.
- The effect of histamine is only transient and lasts for about 15 minutes.
- Kinins dilate capillaries and venules whilst prostaglandins dilate arterioles.
- This produces a more persistent vascular response (24 hours).
- As the vessels dilate, the blood flow reduces.

Cellular phase

- The initial cellular response is from neutrophils.
- As the blood flow reduces, cells move to the sides of the vessels.
- Neutrophils leave the circulation and migrate toward the inflamed area.
- This is followed by the accumulation of macrophages.
- These cellular movements towards the inflammatory site are induced by substances called chemotactic agents.
- Prostaglandin E, some complement factors and lymphokines are known chemotactic agents.

Activated Hageman factor

- The activated Hageman factor stimulates factor XI, leading to fibrin formation.
- This stimulates the kinin cascade, leading to the release of kinins which are vasodilators.
- It also stimulates plasminogen, leading to the formation of plasmin which in turn activates the complement system.

Complement system

- This is a well known cascade system which activates a range of inactive chemicals into their active forms.
- There are two pathways of complement activation, the classical and the alternative pathways; both lead to the same physiological effects.
- The C3a and C5a are called anaphylatoxins. They trigger mast cells and basophils to release vasodilators such as histamine; C5a is also chemotactic.
- Phagocytic cells have receptors for C3b and iC3b that facilitate the adherence of complement coated particles; this allows more effective phagocytosis, and is called opsonization.
- C5b67 is chemotactic with mild cell lysis ability.
- C5b6789 is capable of cell lysis.

Macrophages

- These are derived from monocytes.
- Monocytes enlarge with increase in lysosome numbers and more prominent Golgi apparatus and endoplasmic reticulum.
- Macrophages can be activated by C3b.
- Activated macrophages have increased phagocytotic ability.
- They produce interferon which reduces viral multiplication.
- They stimulate fibroblasts and neutrophils production.
- They produce interleukin-1 which stimulates T-helper cells (*vide infra*).
- They can fuse to form multinucleated giant cells with increased phagocytotic capability.

Immune response

The immune response is specific and targeted at the foreign material. There are two main forms of immune response; the humoral response, which produces antibodies, and the cell-mediated response which produces primed lymphocytes.

Humoral response

Antigen

- An antigen is a substance which is capable of evoking an immune response.
- Most antigens evoke both forms of immune response.
- These responses take place in the lymphoid tissues.
- The products, in the form of antibody and primed lymphocytes, are released into the bloodstream.

Antibodies

- Belong to the immunoglobulin (Ig) plasma proteins.
- Five main classes: IgG, IgM, IgA, IgD and IgE.
- All Ig are composed of one or more similar units.
- Each unit consists of two pairs of identical polypeptide chains, heavy and light chains.

- Each class of Ig has different heavy chains ($\gamma, \mu, \alpha, \delta, \varepsilon$).
- There are only two types of light chains (κ and λ), present in all Ig classes.
- Each unit appears as a 'Y' shaped structure.
- The two 'arms' of each unit are the antigen-binding sites, termed Fab.
- The 'leg' of each unit represent the C-terminal ends of the heavy chains, termed Fc.
- The Fab carries a high level of variability on its N-terminal ends of the light and heavy chains, in order to be able to bind to different antigens.

Immunoglobin classes

There are five main classes of immunoglobins; their differences are summarized in Table 14.1.

Table 14.1 Immunoglobin classes

	IgG	IgM	IgA	IgD	IgE
Main attachment	Polymorph and macrophage	Polymorph and macrophage	Secretion of mucous membrane	Lymphocyte	Mast cell and basophil
Main function	Antitoxins (secondary response)	Antitoxins (primary response)	Activates complement and lysozyme	Lymphocyte surface antigen-receptor	Releases chemicals in mast cells such as histamine
Polymerization	Monomer	Pentamer	Dimer	Monomer	Monomer
Serum concentration (g/l)	8–16	0.5–2	1.4–4	0–0.4	<0.01

Memory effect in the production of antibody

- Exposure to a new antigen generates a primary antibody response.
- Transient and small amount of IgM were produced by day 7.
- Re-exposure to the same antigen generates a secondary antibody response.
- Large amount of IgG is produced by day 4 and the production of IgG persists for weeks.

- This greatly enhanced antibody production is the basis of vaccination.
- Most Ig is produced by plasma cells in lymph nodes, spleen and bone marrow.

Cell-mediated response

Different B lymphocytes carry different surface receptors which are similar to antibodies. When an antigen matches the specific surface receptor on a B lymphocyte, it becomes activated. T lymphocytes are also activated in a similar fashion. These activated cells undergo clonal multiplication and further differentiation. B-cells are converted into plasma cells which produce antibodies, whilst T-cells produce various substances with different properties. Memory cells are also formed during the clonal multiplication. These memory cells are responsible for the memory effects of the increase secondary response on the second exposure to the specific antigen.

T lymphocytes

T lymphocytes are responsible for the specific and non-specific cell-mediated responses. They are subdivided into different groups depending on these surface receptors.

T-cell surface receptors

- Different cell surface molecules have been systematically named by the CD (cluster of differentiation) system.
- Many markers have been identified, the function are unknown for most of the markers (see Table 14.2).
- The CD4 and CD8 markers are best known in view of their role in HIV infections.

Table 14.2 Major T lymphocytes surface markers

Marker	Distribution	Function
CD2	All T-cells	Adherence to target cell
CD3	All T-cells	Signal transduction in antigen recognition
CD4	MHC II restricted T-cells	Binds MHC II molecules
CD8	MHC I restricted T-cells	Binds MHC I molecules

MHC = Major histocompatibility complex

Major histocompatibility complex (MHC)

- MHC is a set of genes located on the short arm of chromosome 6 which code for cell surface glycoprotein.
- MHC plays a major role in self recognition.
- In human, MHC is known as human leucocyte group A (HLA).
- MHC class I antigens are found in all human cells.
- They are coded in the HLA A, B and C regions.
- MHC class II antigens are found on macrophages, Langhans' cells and dendritic cells.
- They are coded in the HLA D regions which can be subdivided into DP, DQ and DR regions.
- The MHC antigens are essential for immune recognition by T lymphocytes which are only able to bind to antigens when they are associated with the MHC molecules.

Subsets of T lymphocytes

T lymphocytes can be subdivided based on their functions. The subsets are summarized in Table 14.3.

Table 14.3 Subsets of T lymphoctyes. NK = natural killer cells, LAK = lymphokine activitated killer cells, K = killer cells.

Subsets	Surface markers	Functions
Helper cells	CD4	Production of lymphokines
Cytotoxic cells	CD8 (90%) CD4 (10%)	Direct cytotoxic effects on virtal infected cells, tumour cells and foreign cells (grafting materials)
Suppressor cells	CD8 (90%) CD4 (10%)	Modulate immune response
MK, LAK, K cells	None	As cytoxic cells but also produce cytokines including γ-inferferon

Cytokines

Cytokines are substances produced by various cells to enhance the immune response. They are named after the cells which produce them. Some of the cytokines also have housekeeping roles in the retina. The most important cytokines are listed in Table 14.4.

Table 14.4 Important cytokines of the immune system

Cytokine	Main source	Main target cells	Main function
Interleukin 1	Monocytes	T & B lymphocytes	Activation
Interleukin 2	T lymphocytes	T lymphocytes	Proliferation and activation
Interleukin 3	T lymphocytes	Stem cells	Increase cell production in bone marrow
Interleukin 4, 5, 6	T lymphocytes	B lymphocytes	Proliferation and activation
Interleukin 7	Stromal cells and fibroblasts	Immature lymphoid cells	Proliferation and differentiation
Interleukin 8	Macrophages	Neutrophils	Chemotaxis
Interleukin 10	T lymphocytes	Mast cells	Growth regulation
Tumour necrosis factor (TNF)	T lymphocytes and macrophages	Macrophages and neutrophils	Activation
Interferon α, β	Leucocytes	Leucocytes	Antiviral effect
Interferon γ	T lymphocytes	Tissue cells	Antiviral effect
Colony stimulating factor (CSF)	T lymphocytes and macrophages	Progenitor cells	Stimulate division and differentiation
Migration inhibition factor (MIF)	T lymphocytes	Macrophages	Migration inhibition
Transforming growth factor β (TGF β)	T lymphocytes and macrophages	T lymphocytes and macrophages	Inhibit activation and growth regulation

Hypersensitivity

Hypersensitivity is defined as an excessive or inappropriate response to an antigenic stimulus. Four types of hypersensitivity are commonly recognized.

- Type I   anaphylactic
- Type II   cytotoxic
- Type III   immune complex
- Type IV   cell-mediated or delayed

Type I: Anaphylactic

- The basic mechanism is mast cell degranulation.
- That is caused by cross-linkage of IgE molecules on mast cell surfaces.
- In a normal immune response, IgM is formed initially, followed by IgG.

- In this type of hypersensitivity, large amounts of IgE are produced in response to certain antigens.
- As the number of IgE on the mast cell surface increases, cross-linkages are possible.
- Degranulated mast cells release histamine, serotonin, heparin, eosinophil and neutrophil chemotactic factors and platelet activating factors.
- These substances lead to vasodilatation and an acute inflammatory response.
- A clinical example is hay fever with allergic eye disease.
- Treatment is by antihistamine and mast cell membrane stabilizers.

Type II: Cytotoxic

- The defect is in the production of antibody that binds to a host cell surface.
- The antigen could be a 'self' membrane receptor or a foreign antigen bound to the cell surface which could be inert.
- For example, autoantibodies against acetylcholine receptors on the muscle end-plate surface, causing myasthenia gravis.
- Once antibody is produced, the host cell 'appears' to be 'foreign' to the immune system.
- The host cell can be destroyed by phagocytes (polymorphs or macrophages), killer lymphocytes and membrane lysis complement complex.
- A special type of type II hypersensitivity occurs in hyperthyroidism (Graves' disease).
- The antibodies stimulate the thyroid stimulating hormone (TSH) receptors on the thyroid cells instead of destroying it; this in turn leads to excess production of thyroid hormones.
- This hypersensitivity reaction is sometimes labelled as type V hypersensitivity by some authors.

Type III: Immune complex

- The basic defect is the formation of soluble immune complex due to a mismatch of antigen to antibody ratio.
- When a soluble antigen combines with antibody, a large aggregate will form.

- These large aggregates can be removed by phagocytes very efficiently.
- However, when there is either antigen excess or antibody excess, smaller and often soluble immune complex is formed.
- They can only be removed slowly by macrophages and not at all by neutrophils.
- These complexes induce an acute inflammatory reaction by activation of the complement systems and macrophages.
- The classical examples are the Arthus' reaction and serum sickness.

Type IV: Cell-mediated or delayed

- As the name suggests, the hypersensitivity is delayed for 24–48 hours.
- It is not associated with antibodies but with activated lymphocytes and macrophages.
- The classical example is the tuberculin response, seen following an intradermal injection of purified protein derivative (PPD) from tubercle bacilli in immune individuals.
- An indurated inflammatory reaction in the skin appears about 24 hours later and persists for a few weeks.
- Normal cell-mediated immune response develops when first exposure of the antigen gives rise to a population of memory cells.
- On the second exposure to the same antigen, these cells are stimulated, start to proliferate and release lymphokines.
- Macrophages and neutrophils are activated as well and a full blown cell-mediated response follows.
- In ophthalmology, the reactivation of herpetic disciform keratitis in the cornea is an example; the damage is most likely caused by cytotoxic T lymphocytes.
- The mainstay of management is in reducing the inflammatory response by topical steroid with prophylactic topical antiviral therapy cover.

Transplantation immunology

- The immune system has the ability to recognize 'self', based on the MHC encoded molecules.

- In humans, the MHC system is called the HLA system.
- A donor graft from another individual will be considered as foreign by the immune system of the recipient.
- It will induce the standard immune response, just like any other antigen.
- In order to minimize the risk of graft rejection, HLA matching is useful.
- As there are a large number of HLA combinations, it is impossible to get a perfect match except from siblings.
- However, some degrees of matching are possible.
- Another approach to reduce rejection rate is by immunosuppression therapy.
- Corticosteroids are most commonly used, and produce non-specific immunosuppression.
- Cytotoxic drugs such as cyclophosphamide, azathioprine, methotrexate and chlorambucil affect all cells of the immune system and other proliferating cells; there is a high incidence of side-effects.
- Cyclosporin is more selective. It is active against T-helper cells and the mode of action is likely to be inhibition of interleukin-2 synthesis and secretion.
- The previous belief that the cornea is a privileged site for transplantation is not completely true; it might be the case when the diseased cornea is not vascularized in cases like corneal dystrophy and keratoconus.
- When the diseased cornea is vascularized, the rejection rate is as high as solid organ transplantation.
- Therefore, clinically, low risk corneal grafting is usually carried out without HLA matching, but high risk corneal grafting such as those with vascularized cornea, herpetic disease and previously failed graft will have HLA matching.
- There is little doubt that HLA matching reduces graft rejection even in the low risk group; however, the benefit is relatively small and may not be cost-effective.

Chapter 15

Ocular pharmacology

In ophthalmology, the most commonly prescribed drugs are topical preparations such as eye drops or ointments. Local injections under the conjunctiva (sub-conjunctival) and the Tenon capsule (sub-Tenon); and periocular injections are other possibilities to deliver high concentrations of medications into the eye.

Systemic preparations are seldom used unless there is no other alternative, in view of the higher risk of systemic side-effects and the poor ocular penetration. On the other hand, systemic absorption from topical therapies can often cause significant systemic effects.

There are four main groups of prescribed therapy:

- Anti-glaucoma therapy.
- Anti-inflammatory therapy.
- Anti-microbial therapy.
- Mydriatic and cycloplegic agents.

Anti-glaucoma therapy

Glaucoma is a relatively common condition. It affects about 1.5–2% of the population. It is difficult to define the condition properly. As a group, it is acceptable to define that glaucoma gives a typical visual field defect with the loss of ganglion cells secondary to a relatively high intraocular pressure for that particular eye. There is evidence that other factors such as optic nerve head circulation, apoptosis and collagen abnormalities play important roles in the pathogenesis of the condition. These factors are beyond the scope of this book and will not be discussed further.

Glaucoma can be divided into primary and secondary. It is then subdivided into open and close angle glaucoma in each group. Primary open angle glaucoma is the most common form of glaucoma and the primary close angle glaucoma (commonly referred as acute glaucoma) requires urgent medical attention.

Aqueous humour is formed in the ciliary body under the control of β (mainly β_2) adrenergic receptors. It escapes the posterior chamber through the pupil into the anterior chamber. It then leaves the angle of the eye through either the trabecular meshwork (conventional pathway) or the uveoscleral pathway (10%).

Topical medications remain the mainstay of management despite a recent move towards early drainage surgery. At the moment, the main goal of all anti-glaucoma therapy is to reduce intraocular pressure. Yet some drops claim to improve optic nerve head circulation and hence reduce the rate of visual field loss.

There are five main groups of anti-glaucoma therapy in current use (see Table 15.1):

- Beta-blockers.
- Miotics.
- Adrenergic agonists.
- Carbonic anhydrase inhibitors.
- Hyperosmotic agents.

Table 15.1 Anti-glaucoma therapy. POAG = primary open angle glaucoma, PACG = primary angle closure glaucoma

	Beta-blockers	Miotics	Adrenergic agonists	Carbonic anhydrase inhibitors	Hyperosmotic agents
Action	Reduce aqueous formation	Increase conventional outflow	Increase uveoscleral outflow	Reduce aqueous formation	Reduce fluid volume in the eye
Mode of action	Blockade of β receptors in ciliary epithelium	Contracts longitudinal fibres of ciliary muscle	α receptor or prostaglandin action	Reduce bicarbonate formation in ciliary processes	Water is drawn by high osmotic pressure
Use in POAG	Treatment of choice	β blockers contraindi-cated	Adjunctive short term therapy	Last resort, role of topical therapy is uncertain	Pre-operatively if IOP is very high
Use in PACG	Acute phase	Acute phase	Contra-indicated	Acute phase	Acute phase
Main problem	Systemic side effects, e.g. broncho-spasm, brady-cardia	Reduce vision and field secondary to miosis	Conjunctival fibrosis – reduce surgical success rate	Profound malaise and confusion in elderly with systemic CAI	Acute diuresis and heart failure
Preparations	Drop	Drop, gel and membranous insert	Drop	Intravenous oral and drop	Intravenous and oral
Commonly used examples	Timolol, levobunolol carteolol betaxolol	Pilocarpine	Adrenaline, dipiverfrine, apraclonidine	Acetazo-lamide, dorzolamide	Mannitol, glycerol and urea

Beta-blockers

These drugs are commonly accepted as the medical treatment of choice, as they do not cause any significant change of visual performance and are least likely to cause conjunctival fibrosis. The main problem is their systemic side-effects, in particular, bronchospasm, bradycardia and heart failure.

They directly compete with adrenaline and noradrenaline for receptor sites in the ciliary body to reduce the aqueous secretion rate and hence the reduction of intraocular pressure (IOP).

Non-selective

- Blocks both β_1 and β_2 receptors.
- The original β blockers.
- Probably still the most commonly prescribed group.
- Examples, timolol and levobunolol.

Selective

- β_1 receptor blockade selectivity is a dose-dependent phenomenon.
- In the eye, the dose should be high enough to block the β_2 receptors as well (75–90% of the β receptor population in the ciliary body are β_2 receptors).
- In the lung, the dose is much smaller and hence there is a lower incidence of bronchospasm, but a high degree of caution is still required in reversible airway diseases.
- Some evidence to suggest that they improve the optic nerve head circulation.
- Clinically, the IOP reduction is less than that of the non-selective β blockers, probably due to their reduced effect on β_2 receptors in the ciliary processes.
- Betaxolol is an example.

Intrinsic sympathomimetic activity (ISA)

- Has partial agonist activity.
- Claimed to be better tolerated systemically.
- Some evidence to suggest that they improve the optic nerve head circulation.

- Clinically, the IOP reduction is similar to the non-selective β blockers.
- On theoretical ground alone, this will be the β blocker of choice.
- Carteolol is an example.

Miotics

Mode of action

- Cholinergic receptors (parasympathetic) are presented in the iris.
- Acetylcholine constricts the pupil by its action on these muscarinic receptors.
- Miotics, such as pilocarpine, act directly on these receptors.
- It is believed that the drug contracts the longitudinal fibres of the ciliary muscle producing traction on the trabecular meshwork allowing aqueous to leave the eye more rapidly.

Clinical indications

- In open angle glaucoma, miotics have been used for many years before the β blockers era.
- In acute glaucoma, the angles of the eye are often narrow; when the pupil is mid-dilated, the resistance for the aqueous to get into the anterior chamber is higher.
- Aqueous collects in the posterior chamber and pushes the peripheral iris forward, causing iris bombé.
- This blocks the angle of the eye and leads to a pressure rise.
- The high pressure causes iris ischaemia and reduces iris movement.
- This vicious cycle leads to an attack of acute glaucoma.

In this situation, miotics reduce the intraocular pressure by pulling the iris flat in reversing the iris bombé and try to break the vicious cycle in addition to the usual mode of action by opening the trabecular meshwork with increase outflow.

In the past, the condition was treated by intensive mitotic therapy in the hope of breaking the vicious cycle. That is difficult to achieve when the pressure remains high and iris ischaemia persists. It is now commonly treated first using other anti-glaucoma therapies such as carbonic anhydrase inhibitor to reduce aqueous production before using miotics.

Main side-effects

- Headache — often transient.
- Reduces visual acuity — miosis and accommodation.
- Reduces visual fields — miosis.
- Pupil rigidity and posterior synechiae — make cataract and retinal surgery difficult.
- Allergy.
- Retinal detachment — uncommon.
- Iris cyst — rare.

Adrenergic agonists

- Adrenaline — non-selective α- and β- adrenergic agonists.
- Dipivefrine — prodrug of adrenaline; it passes through the cornea more rapidly and converts to the active form inside the eye, hence lower concentration is required and less systemic side-effects.
- Apraclonidine — α- adrenergic agonists, in particular α_2 receptors.

Mode of action

Adrenaline and dipivefrine have only a mild IOP reduction effect, and it is understandable that the β- adrenergic action increases the production of aqueous. The mode of action is uncertain, but it is believed that α_2 receptors mediate uveoscleral outflow. Nevertheless, studies have shown that adrenergic agonists increase aqueous outflow through both the conventional trabecular meshwork and the uveoscleral route, and this can be mediated via by endogenous prostaglandin.

Clinical indications

- Mainly used as a second line treatment or as adjunctive therapy.
- Most recent reports disputed the traditional belief in the beneficial effect of adrenaline when used in conjunction with β blockers.
- Nonetheless, there is additional effect of its use with miotics such as pilocarpine.

- Apraclonidine, on the other hand, has adjunctive effects with both β blockers and miotics.
- Apraclonidine can be used to control intraocular pressure rise after cataract surgery and YAG laser capsulotomy.

Main side-effects

- Local allergic response is common with all adrenergic agonists.
- Detrimental effect on the outcome of subsequent glaucoma surgery with adrenaline and dipivefrine, probably due to conjunctival fibrosis induced by the drops. Some surgeons, including the author, will not use these drops unless there is absolutely no alternative, in view of their effect on surgical success.
- Apraclonidine has only a transient IOP lowering effect (lasting for a few months); this tachphylaxis is believed to be due to intraocular receptor changes.
- Blurring of vision secondary to pupil dilatation.
- Cystoid macular oedema in aphakic patients with adrenaline and dipivefrine.
- Systemic side-effects such as hypertension and cardiac arrhythmias are uncommon.

Carbonic anhydrase inhibitors (CAI)

Mode of action

This is the only commonly used systemic anti-glaucoma agent. It can be given either intravenously or orally. In 1995, a topical preparation (dorzolamide) is also available for general use in the UK. Despite the widespread uses, the mode of action is uncertain.

- Carbonic anhydrase is an enzyme to promote the formation of bicarbonate.
- It is abundant in the ciliary body.
- It is believed that the bicarbonate is coupled with the Na/K pump in the ciliary body which secrete aqueous into the posterior chamber.
- CAI block the formation of the bicarbonate and hence reduce aqueous production.

Clinical indications

It is usually used to reduce IOP temporarily until the primary cause of the pressure rise can be treated. Long term use of systemic preparation in primary open angle glaucoma is generally not recommended in view of the high level of systemic side-effects.

The topical preparation can be used as adjunctive therapy to β blockers and miotics. The early results are encouraging but the role of this new preparation in the management of glaucoma will not be established until it is widely used and complications have been documented.

Main side-effects

- Parasthesia of the extremities is almost universal but rarely a problem.
- Profound malaise and lethargy.
- Confusion in elderly.
- Aplastic anaemia — very rare.
- Metabolic acidosis — not usually significant.
- Hypokalaemia — require potassium supplement for long term use.

Hyperosmotic agents

These agents are usually reserved as the last resort to reduce a very high IOP. The action is relatively short-lived and there are potentially life-threatening systemic side-effects.

Mode of action

- Hyperosmotic agents do not or only poorly penetrate the blood–aqueous barrier, yet they are widely distributed in the extracellular space throughout the body.
- Water is drawn from cells and the ocular fluids, including vitreous and aqueous, in order to balance the high osmotic pressure.
- The actual fluid volume of the eye is reduced and hence there is an IOP reduction.
- Commonly used examples include mannitol, glycerol and urea.

Clinical indications

- Reduce IOP immediately pre-operatively.
- In the acute phase of acute glaucoma.

Side-effects

- Acute diuresis — will require catheterization if used pre-operatively.
- Heart failure in particular elderly.
- Rebound cerebral oedema — very rare in ophthalmic use.

Anti-inflammatory therapy

Corticosteroids

Topical steroids

Topical steroid is one of the most commonly used medications in ophthalmology, it is an anti-inflammatory agent.

RELATIVE EFFICACY OF TOPICAL STEROIDS

In descending order for anterior segment inflammation

- Prednisolone acetate 1%
- Dexamethasone 0.1%
- Betamethasone 0.1%
- Prednisolone phosphate 0.5%
- Clobetasone 0.1%
- Fluorometholone 0.1%

COMMON INDICATIONS OF TOPICAL STEROIDS

- Anterior uveitis (iritis).
- Corneal ulcer or inflammation (keratitis).
- Postoperatively in most types of eye surgery.
- Episcleritis.
- Severe allergic conjunctivitis — use with caution.

Systemic steroids

Systemic steroids carry a high rate of systemic side-effects, and its use should be restricted as much as possible.

COMMON INDICATIONS FOR SYSTEMIC STEROIDS IN OPHTHALMOLOGY

- Giant cell arteritis associated with visual loss.
- Severe posterior uveitis or pan-uveitis.
- Pseudotumour of the orbit.
- Pre- and postoperatively in corneal transplant — in selective cases only.
- Optic neuritis — in selective cases only.

Periocular steroids

Local steroid injection in the orbit can be used in some cases of posterior uveitis. The main advantages are better penetration than drops and fewer side-effects than systemic therapy. The disadvantages are the risk of globe penetration during the injection and once it is given, its action can not be stopped or removed. Multiple injections may also be required in most cases.

Anti-inflammatory actions of corticosteroids

Corticosteroids

- Inhibit prostaglandin synthesis (see Figure 15.1).
- Inhibit the increase of capillary dilatation and permeability in inflammation.
- Inhibit the migration of polymorphs and macrophages from the circulation to the inflamed area.
- Modify B-cell response led to reduction of antibody production.
- Inhibit T-cell-mediated macrophages.
- Inhibit eosinophil multiplication.
- Inhibit histamine production.

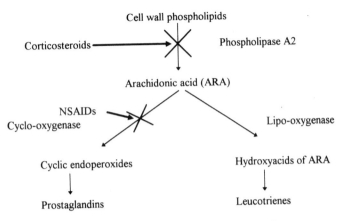

Figure 15.1 Mode of actions of corticosteroids and NSAIDS

Systemic side-effects

- Water retention and weight gain.
- Hypertension.
- Cushing's syndrome (moon face, striae, acne).
- Hypernatraemia (high sodium).
- Hypokalaemia (low potassium).
- Hyperglycaemia (high glucose).
- Osteoporosis.
- Peptic ulceration.
- Adrenal suppression.
- Muscle wasting.
- Confusion.

Ocular side-effects

- Cataracts, in particular, posterior subcapsular cataract.
- Raised intraocular pressure in 'steroid responder' (*vide infra*).
- Exacerbates viral keratitis, in particular, herpetic dendritic ulcers.
- Allergic conjunctivitis — usually associated with the preservatives in the eyedrop.
- Peripheral corneal thinning and scleral melting — rare.

Corticosteroids and steroid responders

- Steroid responders are patients who develop high intraocular pressure (>30 mmHg) after a course of topical steroid.
- The response does not usually occur until at least 2 weeks after commencing the therapy.
- Stronger steroids such as dexamethasone and betamethasone have significantly more hypertensive effect than weaker steroids like fluorometholone.
- About 5% of the population are steroid responders.
- However, >90% of glaucoma patients are steroid responders.
- Diabetic retinopathy and high myopia are also high risk groups.
- The exact mechanism is unknown, but it is believed to be secondary to swelling of cells in the trabecular meshwork causing reduction of aqueous outflow.

Non-steroidal anti-inflammatory drugs (NSAID)

- NSAIDs inhibit prostaglandin synthesis (see Figure 15.1).
- Prostaglandins are normally released in inflammatory responses and are involved in causing pain, redness and swelling.
- NSAIDs block the conversion of arachidonic acid to cyclic endoperoxides by inhibition of cyclo-oxygenase.
- In the eye, prostaglandins are released during intraocular surgery which can cause pupillary constriction and make the operation more difficult to perform.

Side-effects

- Gastric irritation.
- Increase bleeding time.

Clinical ophthalmic uses

- Posterior scleritis — orally.
- Postoperative uses in retinal detachment surgery and vitreo–retinal surgery — orally.
- Postoperative uses in cataract and glaucoma surgery — topically.
- Inhibition of intraoperative miosis during cataract surgery — topically.

Other anti-inflammatory agents

- Topical preparations of anti-histamines, sodium cromoglycate and lodoxamide are available for allergic conjunctivitis and vernal catarrh.
- The efficacy of anti-histamine is relatively restricted in chronic allergic eye diseases.
- Both sodium cromoglycate and lodoxamide are membrane stabilizers and hence reduce the release of histamine and other inflammatory agents from mast cells.
- Lodoxamide is claimed to reduce chemotaxis (attraction of inflammatory cells).

Anti-microbial therapy

There are many different types of antibiotics and anti-viral therapies. It is inappropriate to cover all of them. The following is a selection of the most commonly used preparations in ophthalmology. Fungal infections of the eye are fortunately rare and their treatment is complex. It is not covered here.

Antibiotics

Chloramphenicol

In 1995, chloramphenicol is still the most commonly used topical antibiotic in Britain. As a broad spectrum antibiotic, it remains the treatment of choice for superficial ocular infection. Its use in the US and some European countries has been reduced substantially in view of the potential fatal side-effect of aplastic anaemia. In general, both ophthalmologists and haematologists in Britain do not think the risk is high enough to restrict its use in the topical form. However, its use in systemic form is inappropriate unless there is no alternative.

- First isolated in Streptomycetes from soil in Venezuela and a compost heap in Illinois.
- The commercial form is manufactured synthetically.
- It blocks peptidyl transferase which links amino acids in growing peptide chain, thus stops the process of bacterial growth.
- It is a strictly bacteriostatic agent in the therapeutic range.

- It is a broad spectrum antibiotic against both Gram positive and Gram negative bacteria.
- Resistance strains of Gram negative cocci, *H. influenzae* and Staphylococci are present.
- This resistance is usually caused by a few different types of acetylase enzymes.

SIDE-EFFECTS

- Ocular and systemic side-effects of topical chloramphenicol are very uncommon.
- The risk of developing aplastic anaemia is said to be 13 times higher if systemic chloramphenicol is given.
- There is no concrete evidence that topical therapy can cause aplastic anaemia as well, it is theoretically possible and there have been some case reports.
- Optic neuritis has been described in children with prolonged therapy.

CLINICAL OPHTHALMIC USES

- It is the treatment of choice in superficial ocular infection.
- It is commonly used as a prophylactic antibiotic after corneal foreign body removal and viral conjunctivitis.
- It is commonly used as a pre- and postoperative prophylactic antibiotics in both extraocular and intraocular surgery.

Aminoglycosides

- As a group, they are polycationic compounds which are either naturally occurring or semi-synthetic.
- They block protein synthesis and cause misreading of mRNA on the ribosome; unlike chloramphenicol, they are bactericidal agents.
- The main action is against Gram negative aerobic bacteria and some Gram positive Staphylococcus. Some strains of *Pseudomonus aeruginosa* is also sensitive to aminoglycosides.
- They have bactericidal synergy with β-lactams agents (pencillins and cephalosporins).

SIDE-EFFECTS

- Systemic use is restricted in view of the high risk of ototoxicity (hearing loss) and nephrotoxicity (kidney failure).
- Neuromuscular blockade in high dosage. It is not clinically significant except in patients receiving muscle relaxants or anaesthesia, or in myasthenia gravis patients.
- Local irritation and allergy response are common (about 10%) with topical preparations; some patients might require alternative therapy.

CLINICAL OPHTHALMIC USES

- Topical use of gentamicin, neomycin and tobramycin are common in superficial ocular infections including cornea ulcers.
- Combined steroids with neomycin preparations are used commonly in postoperative patients to improve compliance.
- Gentamicin is commonly given at the end of intraocular surgery subconjunctivally; it might, however, cause conjunctival necrosis and very rarely retinal toxicity.
- Aminoglycoside is added by some surgeons in the irrigation fluid for cataract and vitreo-retinal surgery to reduce postoperative infection (endophthalmitis).
- Amikacin can also be used as intravitreal injection as its retinal toxicity is less than other aminoglycosides in severe intraocular infection such as endophthalmitis.

Fluoroquinolones

This drug is a modification of the old quinolones antibiotic group (e.g. nalidixic acid) by introduction of fluorine into the 6-position of the molecule. This reduces the frequency of the CNS side-effects significantly.

- Ciprofloxacin is a synthetic fluoropiperazinyl quinolone and the prime example of this group of antibiotics.
- It inhibits the DNA gyrase which is essential for nucleic acid synthesis, bacteria cell death is rapid with this process being inhibited.
- It is a broad spectrum bactericidal antibiotic against both Gram positive and Gram negative bacteria.

- Its action against Pseudomonus species especially *P. aeruginosa*, *H. influenzae*, and Gram positive cocci (Staphylococci and Streptococci) is most welcome in the ophthalmology practice.
- It can penetrate the non-inflamed eye with a normal oral dosage.
- Resistance in Britain is uncommon in 1995. There have been reports in the spread of resistant strains of *Staph. aureus* in the US. Interestingly, some new patients were found to be colonized by the resistant strains without having ciprofloxacin themselves.

SIDE-EFFECTS

- Gastrointestinal disturbance (4–10%).
- CNS disturbances as in quinolones (1–2%).
- Pseudomembranous colitis — uncommon.
- Potentiation of the action of theophylline.

CLINICAL OPHTHALMIC USES

- Corneal ulcers, in particular Pseudomonas ulcers (topical).
- Endophthalmitis (oral or intravenous).

Cephalosporins

- This is a large and expanding group of antibiotics based in cephalosporin C which was originally found in the fermentation products of *Cephalosporium acremonium*.
- The fused ring system of cephalosporins is similar to that of penicillins and a β-lactam ring is present.
- Most second and third generation of cephalosporins have resistance against β-lactamases (a main source of resistance for penicillins) and a wider bactericidal spectrum.
- They inhibit bacterial cell wall synthesis.
- The main action is against Gram positive bacteria; however, the newer drugs have significant action against Gram negative bacteria.
- Synergy action against bacteria with aminoglycosides (which cover most Gram negative organisms) makes them a popular combination for initial treatment of severe ocular infection before culture results are available.

SIDE-EFFECTS

- Cephalosporins are usually well tolerated.
- Cross-allergic reaction with penicillin (about 5–10 % of pencillin allergic patients show reaction to cephalosporins) — it is common practice not to use them in penicillin allergic patients unless there is no alternative.

CLINICAL OPHTHALMIC USES

- Corneal ulcers (topical) — usually combined with aminoglycosides.
- Immediate postoperatively in intraocular surgery (subconjunctival).
- Endophthalmitis (topical, oral or intravenous).

Fusidic acid

- A fermentation product of *Fusidium coccineum*.
- It forms a complex with an elongation factor and hence stop protein synthesis.
- Its main action is against Gram positive bacteria and some action against Gram negative cocci.
- Resistance is uncommon.

CLINICAL OPHTHALMIC USES

- The development of fusidic acid in a gel preparation to allow a twice-daily regime made it a popular choice for superficial ocular infection.

Tetracyclines

- A group of natural products derived from *Streptomyces* species.
- Some are natural products and others are semi-synthetics.
- They inhibit protein synthesis by attaching to the 30S ribosomal subunits.
- The main action is against Gram positive bacteria and some action against Gram negative bacteria.
- They are also active against Chlamydia and *P. acnes*.
- They decrease fatty acids and increase triglycerides in skin surface lipids.

SIDE-EFFECTS

- Gastrointestinal disturbances.
- Glossitis.
- Pruritus ani, vulvitis and vaginitis.

   Deposit in teeth and bone — not to be used in pregnancy and in children.

CLINICAL OPHTHALMIC USES

- Chlamydia infections, include trachoma.
- Lid margin disease — in view of their ability to alter surface lipids.

Anti-viral therapy

Acyclovir

- A synthetic acyclic purine nucleoside analogue.
- Active against herpes simplex type 1 and 2, simian herpes virus B and herpes zoster viruses.
- Acyclovir monophosphate (inactive) is converted to acyclovir triphosphate (active agent) by viral thymidine kinase which is only presented in the herpes-infected cells.
- The active agent inhibits herpes virus DNA polymerase and a DNA chain terminator, thus blocking viral replication.

SIDE-EFFECTS

- Nausea and vomiting.
- Encephalopathy — uncommon.
- Bone marrow depression — uncommon.
- Abnormal liver function — uncommon.

OPHTHALMIC CLINICAL USES

- Herpes simplex keratitis (dendritic ulcers).
- Ophthalmic zoster in the early stage.
- Prophylaxis in a previously herpetic infected eye for topical steroids used, such as after corneal grafting for herpetic disciform scar.
- Acute retinal necrosis.

Ganciclovir

- A synthetic nucleoside analogue.
- It is phosphorylated to the monophosphate in infected cells more rapidly than in non-infected cells. It is then further metabolized to the triphosphate active form by cellular enzymes.
- Herpes simplex and herpes zoster viruses induce their own thymidine kinase and effectively phosphorylate ganciclovir.
- Cytomegalovirus (CMV) and Epstein–Barr virus do not encode the enzyme and the phosphorylate mechanism is uncertain, yet there is a ten fold increase of the triphosphate compound in the CMV infected cells as compared with the non-infected cells.
- Oral bioavailability is poor and hence intravenous use is usually required. Intravitreal use is also possible.
- It is only a virustatic agent and hence life-long maintenance therapy is required.

SIDE-EFFECTS

- Bone marrow suppression causing neutropenia — concomitant use with zidovudine in AIDS patients is usually impossible.
- CNS effects — convulsions, dizziness, headaches.
- Gastrointestinal effects — nausea, vomiting, diarrhoea.
- Abnormal liver function.

CLINICAL OPHTHALMIC USES

- Cytomegalovirus (CMV) retinitis.

Foscarnet

- A synthetic non-nucleoside pyrophosphate analogue.
- It inhibits the DNA polymerases of herpes simplex, cytomegalovirus and Epstein–Barr virus.
- Intravenous and intravitreal preparations are available.
- Like ganciclovir, it is only a virustatic agent and hence life-long maintenance therapy is required.

SIDE-EFFECTS

● Nausea and vomiting.
● Renal failure — this is the limiting factor for its use.
● Hypocalcaemia.
● Headache.

CLINICAL OPHTHALMIC USES

● Cytomegalovirus (CMV) retinitis.

Mydriatic and cycloplegic agents

Acetylcholinergic antagonists

● Atropine and related compounds produce a direct antagonist effect on muscarinic cholinergic receptors.
● They cause pupillary dilatation (mydriasis) and abolish accommodation (cycloplegia).

Side-effects

● Dry mouth.
● Constipation.
● Blurred vision.
● Can precipitate angle closure glaucoma — rare.

Clinical ophthalmic uses

● Pupillary dilatation for fundal examination and surgery.
● Cycloplegic refraction, especially in children.
● Anterior segment inflammation, including iritis, to relieve painful pupillary spasm and reduce posterior synechiae (iris-lens attachment).
● Amblyopia treatment by inducing blurred vision on the 'good' eye when patching cannot be tolerated.

Relative potencies and durations of action in descending order

● Atropine (7 days).
● Homatropine (24–48 h).

- Cyclopentolate (12–24 h).
- Tropicamide (3–4 h) — it has virtually no cycloplegic action hence inappropriate for cycloplegic refraction.

Sympathomimetics

- Phenylephrine is the only commonly used sympathomimetic.
- It is an α-adrenergic receptor agonist.
- It causes pupillary dilatation without cycloplegia.
- It also causes vasoconstriction.

Side-effects

- Pigment release in the anterior chamber.
- Blurred vision.
- Can precipitate angle closure glaucoma — rare.
- Hypertension and bradycardia.

Clinical ophthalmic uses

- Pupillary dilatation for fundal examination and surgery.
- It can be obtained without prescription for undiagnosed red eye — this indication is not recommended.

Chapter 16

Basic genetics

It is amazing that most of our cells carries a copy of our genetic identity yet the expression of that could not be more difference in different cells. Genetic factors are implicated in many diseases.

Some of these are well known hereditary diseases such as retinitis pigmentosa. The mode of transmission follows Mendelian laws. In others, a positive family history increases the risk of developing certain diseases, such as glaucoma. Whether the disease is carried by a combination of genes or the trigger lies in the environment is highly uncertain. Furthermore, the understanding of mitochondrial DNA opens a new approach in research towards certain diseases such as Leber's optic atrophy.

Molecular genetics in ophthalmic diseases is an exciting new area. Since the discovery of rhodopsin mutation in autosomal dominant retinitis pigmentosa, a number of other interesting factors have been found. With the improved understanding of the disease process, gene therapy is getting closer to reality. This is probably the most interesting and exciting field in ophthalmology. This view might be biased in view of my own research interest.

Chromosomal disorders

- Chromosomes contain DNA.
- Human has 46 chromosomes, 22 pairs with two sex chromosomes (X, Y).
- Incidence of chromosomal disorders is about 0.6%.

Numerical abnormalities

There are an abnormal number of chromosomes.

Triploidy

- A total of 69 chromosomes.
- Always fatal.
- Due to failure of meiosis or 2 spermatozoa fertilizing one egg.

Trisomy

- A total of 47 chromosomes.
- Chromosome pair failed to separate and move together to the same pole of cell due to non-disjunction in meiosis.
- Incidences increase with increasing maternal age, perhaps as a failure of female meiosis.
- Trisomy 21 — Down's syndrome.
- Trisomy 18 — Edward syndrome.
- Trisomy 13 — Patau syndrome.

Monosomy

- Only 45 chromosomes.

- Classical example is Turner syndrome 44 XO.
- That is 44 chromosomes with only 1 X chromosome.

Structural abnormalities

This implies a structural change of the chromosome.

Translocation

- Transfer of DNA between chromosomes.
- Requiring breakage of both chromosomes with repair in an abnormal arrangement.
- If no loss or gain of DNA — clinically normal — called balanced translocation.
- At risk of having chromosomally abnormal offspring (unbalanced translocation).

Deletion and duplication

- Deletion or duplication of a segment of chromosomal material.
- Deletion is usually more harmful.
- Deletion of short arm of chromosome 11 (11p) is associated with aniridia (absence of iris).

Single gene disorders

- Each gene occupies a specific locus on a specific chromosome.
- The autosomal genes are arranged in pairs with one maternal and one paternal origin.
- If the gene pair is identical, it is called homozygous, if not, heterozygous.
- Abnormal gene which arises by mutation may not interfere with normal cell function.
- Trait is a disease gene or genes which determines the characteristics (>4000 traits were found in humans).
- Incidence of single gene disorders is about 1–1.5% of livebirths.
- Have a high rate of morbidity and mortality with high risk to siblings.

Autosomal dominant (AD) conditions

- AD trait manifests the trait (disease) even in heterozygote state.
- One of the parents always carries the abnormal gene.
- Variable expressivity and incomplete penetrance is common in AD diseases.
- It is important to know the difference in risk estimation for genetic counselling.
- Variable expressivity is present if individuals are affected to a different degree of severity.
- Incomplete penetrance is present if not all carriers manifest the disease.
- Familial dominant drusen, Stickler syndrome and Marfan's syndrome can be transmitted as AD conditions.
- Equal frequency and severity in each sex.
- As shown in Figure 16.1, half of the offsprings will carry the defected gene.
- However, if the penetrance is, for example, 80%.
- The risk of developing the disease will be 50% of 80% = 40%.

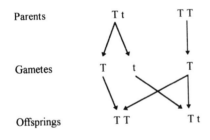

Figure 16.1 Autosomal dominant conditions. T = normal gene: t = defective gene: TT = normal: Tt = heterozygous (i.e. disease)

Autosomal recessive (AR) conditions

- AR trait manifests only in homozygote state.
- Oculocutaneous albinism, Leber's congenital amaurosis and Stargardt's macular dystrophy can be transmitted as AR conditions.

Parents

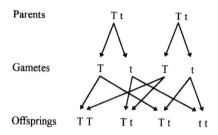

Figure 16.2 Autosomal recessive conditions. T = normal gene: t = defective gene: TT = normal: Tt = heterozygous state (i.e. carrier): tt = homozygous state (i.e. disease)

- Equal frequency and severity in each sex.
- Assuming both parents are not affected and hence carriers of the disease, the risk of having an affected child will be 1 in 4 as shown in Figure 16.2. By chance, 50% of the offsprings will be carriers.

Comparison between AD and AR conditions

The main differences between AD and AR conditions are summarized in Table 16.1.

Table 16.1 Comparison between AD and AR conditions

	Autosomal dominant	*Autosomal recessive*
Disease expressed	Heterozygote	Homozygote
Risk to siblings	1 in 2	1 in 4
Risk to offsprings	1 in 2	Very low
Expressivity	Variable	Constant in a family
Pedigree pattern	Vertical	Horizontal
Other factors	Increase paternal age	Consanguinity

X-linked recessive conditions

- Over 280 X-linked conditions have been described.
- Males only have one X chromosome from the maternal side.
- Hence, no male to male transmission.
- No risks to male offsprings, but all female offsprings are carriers.
- Colour blindness and choroidoraemia can be transmitted as XL recessive conditions.

X-linked dominant and Y-linked inheritance

- Very uncommon.
- Male sufferers are more severely affected than their female counterpart in XL dominant.

Multifactorial inheritance

- Many conditions are determined by the summation of the effects of many genes at different loci coupled with environmental factors.
- There is an increased risk to relatives but not as high compared with the Mendelian mode of inheritance.
- Glaucoma and age-related macular degeneration are believed to be transmitted by multifactorial inheritance.

Mitochondrial inheritance

- Human mitochondria have their own DNA (mDNA).
- Mitochondria are present only in the cytoplasm.
- Therefore, spermatozoa carry no cytoplasm at the fertilization stage.
- All mDNA is transmitted from the maternal side in the egg.
- Leber's optic atrophy can be transmitted by mitochondrial inheritance.
- This mode of inheritance cannot totally explain the bias towards male sufferers in Leber's optic atrophy.

Molecular genetics

Structure of DNA

- DNA consists of two long chains of sugar deoxyribose and phosphate residues forming a double helix.
- These chains are formed by the loss of two water molecules to condense a phosphoric acid residue with two deoxyribose molecules, one being attached through its 5-hydroxyl and the other through its 3-hydroxyl.

- Hence, each chain has a 3′ end and a 5′ end.
- Each deoxyribose residue in the chain is substituted by either a purine or pyrimidine base.
- The purine bases are adenine and guanine, whilst the pyrimidine bases are thymine and cytosine.
- Watson and Crick were first to suggest that there is complementary anti-parallel base pairing on the two chains in the double helix.
- Adenine is always paired with thymine, whilst guanine is always paired with cytosine.
- Therefore, the two chains are complementary and specific for each other.
- An example is shown in Figure 16.3.

3′CGATCGA............ATTCCGG5′
5′GCTAGCT............TAAGGCC3′

Figure 16.3 DNA sequence

Genetic coding

- The DNA code the precise information for protein synthesis.
- In practice, only one strand in the double helix is used for protein synthesis.
- A base triplet (three bases in a DNA chain) codes an amino acid (called codon).
- As there are four different purines and pyrimidine bases, there are 64 possible combinations.
- Since there are only 20 different amino acids, some amino acids are encoded by more than one base triplet.

DNA finger printing

- Restriction enzymes cleave double stranded DNA in or near a particular DNA sequence of nucleotides.
- In other words, they cut the DNA chains into many fragments at specific points.
- There are now more than 300 different restriction enzymes.

- Digesting DNA from a specific source using a particular set of restriction enzymes will produce the same reproducible collection of DNA fragments each time.
- The DNA fragments are divided by electrophoresis based on the theory that smaller molecules travel faster than larger ones.
- A 'map' with a larger number of bands can be seen.
- As our DNA is unique, the DNA map is also unique; this is the basic principle of DNA finger printing.

Polymerase chain reaction (PCR)

- It is difficult not to mention molecular genetics without mentioning PCR.
- PCR can be used to produce vast quantities of a DNA fragment provided that the base pair sequence of that region is known.
- The technique involves synthesizing two oligonucleotide primers complementary to the DNA flanking a particular DNA sequence of interest.
- The source DNA is denatured by heat, allowing the two chains to be separated.
- The primers attach themselves to the DNA chains.
- DNA polymerase assists the extension of the primer and forms another copy of the DNA sequence of interest.
- The process is repeated again with reheating and cooling; in each cycle, the number of the DNA sequence of interest is doubled.
- The PCR process can now be carried out automatically by machine.
- In theory, DNA analysis is possible even from a single cell using PCR technique.

Basic principles of gene therapy

- 'Foreign' DNA can be inserted into the host cells to alter its function.
- Host DNA can be cleaved by specific restriction enzyme.
- A foreign DNA can be inserted into the cleaved site as long as the restriction enzyme can cleave the foreign DNA to give a free fragment.

Host DNA

...GCGCAATTCGATC...
...CGCGTTAAGCTAG...

Cleaved host DNA

...GCGC   AATTCGATC...
...CGCGTTAA   GCTAG...

Foreign DNA

..GCAATTATCGTTAACCC.
..CGTTAATAGCAATTGGG.

Cleaved foreign DNA

..GC   *AATTATCG*   TTAATCC.
..CGTTAA   *TAGCTTAA*   AGG.

Final host DNA

...GCGC*AATTATCG*AATTCGATC...
...CGCGTTAA*TAGCTTAA*GCTAG...

Figure 16.4 Illustration of DNA insertion

- An illustration is given in Figure 16.4, only four base pairs are inserted into the host DNA in this illustration; in real life a much longer chain is inserted.
- The new chain can be used to produce a new protein which can be the defective protein in a hereditary disease.
- This technique is also used to allow sheep producing human insulin in their milk.

Section D
Investigations and laser

Fluorescein and its use

Sodium fluorescein is commonly used in ophthalmology. It carries an interesting property that it can be excited by one colour of light and emits another colour of light. This special property is used extensively in fundal fluorescein angiography (FFA) which has a major role in the study of retinal diseases.

Properties of sodium fluorescein

- Fluorescein is the emission of energy at one wavelength (colour) in response to irradiation by a shorter wavelength.
- Sodium fluorescein is highly water soluble.
- Excitation wavelength is about 490 nm.
- This wavelength causes a momentary shift of its molecular structure, when it returns to its normal state, kinetic energy emits as light.
- When it returns to its normal state, kinetic energy emits as light.
- Emits a wavelength of about 520 nm.
- However, in blood, excited by 465 nm and emits at 525 nm.
- Binds with albumin (70–80%).
- Equally distributed throughout blood within 3–5 min.

- Rapidly eliminated — mainly by kidney.
- Majority of dye is eliminated within 1 hour after intravenous injection.

Clinical uses of fluorescein in ophthalmology

- Fundal fluorescein angiography.
- Detection of corneal epithelial defects.
- Applanation tonometry.
- Tear film assessment.
- Hard contact lens fitting.
- Seidel's test for corneal wound leakage.
- Test of nasolacrimal drainage system.
- Anterior segment angiography.

Fundal fluorescein angiography (FFA)

Fundal fluorescein angiography is one of the most commonly used techniques in the study of retinal disease. In the choroid, there are no tight junctions; fluorescein can then leak out and produces the choroidal flush. The outer retinal barrier in the RPE cells stops it from getting into the retina.

As mentioned before, fluorescein is heavily bound to the protein. It does not normally leak out of the retinal vessels which form the inner blood–retinal barrier. Any leakage implies an abnormality. FFA is divided into different phases.

Different phases of FFA

1. Arm — retinal circulation time (8–10 s).

2. Background choroidal flush.

- Filling of choroiocapillaries via the posterior ciliary arteries.
- Patchy filling at posterior pole initially.
- This reflects leakage of choroidal vessels.
- Retinal pigment epithelium (RPE) acts as a barrier to leakage from choroid to retina.

3. Arterial phase (1 s later after choroidal flush).

● Filling of the arteries only.

4. Capillary phase (arterial–venous phase).

● Complete arterial and capillary filling with venous lamina flow.

5. Venous phase

● Complete venous filling.

6. Recirculation phase (complete between 3 and 5 min).

● Early leakage or staining occurs at this stage.

7. Elimination phase (30–60 min).

● Late staining and residual leakage of dye is seen.

Causes of hyperfluorescence

● Atrophy of RPE cells (window effect) — the RPE cells normally attenuate the emitted light of the fluorescein from the choroid, if there are RPE atrophy, the fluorescein can be seen more clearly.
● Dye in subretinal space.
● Dye in RPE detachment.
● Dye leakage of retinal vessels, e.g. in diabetic retinopathy.
● Dye leakage from choroidal or retinal new vessels.
● Dye leakage in optic nerve head, e.g. in papilloedema.
● Staining of tissues by dye, e.g. drusen.

Causes of hypofluorescence

● Masking by abnormal materials, e.g. blood, melanin, hard exudate.
● Ischaemia retina causing capillary drop-out.
● Ischaemia choroid.
● Atrophy of vascular tissues, e.g. in myopia.

Side-effects of fluorescein

- Yellow discoloration of skin and dark urine.
- Nausea — 15–30 s after injection, subsides within 1 min.
- Itching.
- Syncope.
- Laryngeal oedema and even anaphylactic shock — very rare.

Chapter 18

Visual field testing

The normal visual field extends about 60 degrees superiorly, 75 degrees inferiorly, 100 degrees temporally and 60 degrees nasally. Using a small target or a dim light, the visual field will be more restricted. This is due to the sensitivity to the target decreases in all directions away from the point of fixation. The visual field is really a three-dimensional structure.

The best description of the visual field was by Traquair in 1931. He described the visual field as a hill or island of vision in a sea of blindness. Just like mapping the hills, the visual field can be documented in a two-dimensional graph.

The contours of equal sensitivity (as compared with height in map) are called isoptres. Using certain standardized target sizes and illuminations, the visual field can be presented as a map with concentric ovals. Like the map, the variability of sensitivity is indirectly shown by the variability in spacing of the isoptres. In other word, when the 'slope of vision' is steep as in neurological field loss, the isoptre lines will be very close to each other.

Static and kinetic visual field testing — basic principles

In static testing, targets of various sizes and intensities are presented at the same location. It determines the presence and depth of a scotoma (visual field loss).

In kinetic testing, a series of targets of fixed size and intensity are moved from the nonseeing to seeing areas of the visual field. The foci identified kinetically are corresponding points at each sensitivity level that is on the same isoptres.

Tangent screen

The tangent screen, like a Bjerrum screen, is a flat screen mounted on the wall. It is particularly useful in neuro-ophthalmology practice when the visual field loss tends to be more dense and large.

Advantages of the tangent screen

- Cheap.
- Convenient.
- Simple to use.
- Fast.

Disadvantages of the tangent screen

- Non-standardized test parameters such as the background illumination.
- Require constant monitoring of fixation by the examiner.
- The target intensities cannot be changed.
- Visual field testing is generally limited to the central 30 degrees.
- Evaluation of patient reliability is purely subjective.

Arc perimetry

● A rotatable semicircular band with a radius of about 33 cm serving as the background on which stimulus lights are presented.

● Test parameters are still non-standardized.

● Can be tested beyond 30 degrees.

Bowl perimetry

● Goldmann bowl perimetry is still one of the most commonly used manual visual field test machines.

● The bowl measures 33 cm in radius and extends 95 degrees to each side of fixation.

● Stimulus size and intensity can each be varied giving a measure in apostilbs.

● The testing distance and background illumination is standardized.

● Both kinetic and static perimetry can be carried out with Goldmann.

Computerized automated static perimetry

The move towards computerized automated perimetry is not without reason. It is very simple to use and more reliable to reproduce. Some machines can even provide a report with the numeric figures and the probability index of abnormalities. Static bowl perimetry is the norm, as kinetic perimetry demands control of the speed and direction of movement making hardware design more difficult.

Advantages

● Test administration is more standardized and hence more reproducible.

● Less subjective input from the examiner, hence less variability.

● Automated fixation monitoring improves reliability.

● Patient dependability may be quantitated and statistically assessed.

- Ability of data storage.
- Allow for sequential fields analysis.
- Less experience and training required for the examiner.

Disadvantages

- Much more expensive.
- Requires mechanical servicing.
- Full field threshold takes a long time to do, causing patient fatigue with possible unreliable results.
- Requires higher degree of co-operation from the patient.
- Slow response time by the patient can cause unreliable results.
- Not suitable for advance field loss.

In order to understand and interpret computerized visual field analysis, some of the basic concepts will be discussed.

The concept of threshold

- Threshold is defined as the minimal intensity of light at which a stimulus is perceived by the eye at a specific location in the field of vision.
- Suprathreshold is any stimulus brighter than threshold.
- Infrathreshold is any stimulus weaker than threshold.

Light intensities

- Apostilb (asb) is an absolute measurement of light intensity reflected from a surface.
- It is commonly used in manual perimetry.
- Variations in presented light intensities are not perceived by the eye in a linear manner but on a relative scale.
- In computerized perimetry, the decibel (dB) scale is used to express retinal sensitivities.
- Decibel scale is a logarithmic scale based on the maximum stimulus a perimeter may produce.
- Decibels are the reciprocal of log intensity in apostilbs.
- The higher the decibel value, the dimmer the stimulus (i.e. lower apostilb value).

Hardware consideration

- The bowl radius in the Humphrey field analyser (one of the most commonly used computerized perimetry) is 33 cm, as in the Goldmann. Corrective lens is required to compensate for the accommodation required.

- Background illumination varies in different machines.

- The dimmer background allows the machine to present relatively brighter stimuli to the eye with respect to the background light which is useful for patients with markedly reduced sensitivity.

- The disadvantages include the risk of shifting retinal sensitivity to the scotopic range and the effect of media opacities may be more pronounced.

Testing patterns and strategies

- The examiner has to decide the pattern and strategy to use for an individual patient.

- Testing pattern refers to the area of visual field to be examined. For instance, the central 30 degrees or central 24 degrees and so on.

- Specific patterns to look for nasal step and temporal wedge in glaucoma and vertical meridians in neurological cases can be used. This is often offered as specific options in the computerized perimetry. For instance, a 24–2 program in Humphrey is referred to central 24 degrees with glaucoma pattern.

- Suprathreshold screening field can identify gross field loss very quickly; the disadvantage includes missing subtle field defects.

- Threshold determination field provides the most accurate information but is time-consuming.

Threshold determination strategy

- A stimulus brighter than the patient's expected threshold is presented.

- If it is seen, stimuli of successively reduced intensity are presented until the stimulus is not seen.

- Then stimuli of increasing intensity are presented until it is seen again.

- The threshold is the average of the cross-over points.

Evaluation of the result

In most computerized perimetry, a printout of results is provided. In general, there is a diagrammatic representation of the field, reliability indices and global indices.

Diagrammatic representation

- Black spots to represent dense field loss.
- Variable scale of grey spots to represent variable degree of reduction in retinal sensitivity.
- White spots for normal sensitivity.

Reliability indices

- Fixation loss — it is assumed that if fixation is maintained, the blind spot should not move. Hence if a spot within the previous determined blind spot can be seen by the patient during the field test, it is an indication of fixation loss and hence less reliable.
- A false positive response is recorded if the patient signals the presence of a stimulus when none has been presented. High value indicates poor reliability.
- False negative response is recorded if a superthreshold stimulus is not registered by the patient, it is usually an indication of poor reliability. However, glaucoma patients have been shown to have a higher rate of false negative respond.

Global indices

- Mean deviation (MD) is the difference between mean sensitivity obtained and that of expected for the patient's age. A high value can be caused by media opacities, poor vision, miosis and unreliability.
- Pattern standard deviation (PSD) is a reflection of the regional non-uniformity of a visual field. A high value suggests a localized defect.
- Short term fluctuation (SF) is a measure of the variability of threshold sensitivity at a given tested point during the same examination. A high value is associated with glaucoma patients, unreliable patients and those with high value of mean deviation.

- Corrected pattern standard deviation (CPSD) takes into account the effect of short term fluctuation (SF) on pattern standard deviation (PSD). This is more sensitive to the presence of localized defects, correcting for coexisting diffuse fluctuations.
- A probability value for each index is often given to indicate the probability of true deviation from normal.

Clinical points

- Computerized perimetry requires a high degree of co-operation from the patients. There is no point in asking for this type of perimetry for a confused or frail patient.
- The instruction is quite complicated for many patients. There should be a 'learning field test session' before a formal field analysis.
- The best way to appreciate the patient's difficulties of visual field testing is to have the test done on yourself.

Chapter 19

Electrodiagnostic techniques

Electroretinography (ERG)

The standard ERG (Table 19.1) is a recording of electrical signals from the retina elicited by a flash of light. The response is believed to be caused by a transient movement of ions in the extracellular space induced by the light.

Table 19.1 Normal values in flash ERG

Normal values	a-wave	b-wave	Oscillatory potentials
Scotopic	> 200 μV	> 300 μV	> 4 in number (~8–10 μV)
Photopic	> 30 μV	> 60 μV	> 3 in number (4–5 μV)
30 Hz flicker (cone response)			

Standard flash ERG

● Measures the initial 200 ms.

● Two predominant responses; a-wave and b-wave.

● a-wave is the initial downgoing deflection — photoreceptor response.

● b-wave is the upgoing deflection — Muller and bipolar cell response.

● Oscillatory potential is seen mainly on b-wave — amacrine cell response.

● Ganglion cells play no role at all.

● Hence, inner layer and optic nerve damage — normal flash ERG.

● ERG is a mass response of the whole retina.

● Hence, localized lesion in retina will have normal flash ERG.

Methods

● Light stimulus is delivered via a full field bowl (ganzfeldt).

● ERG is recorded directly from the eye via a corneal contact lens or more recently by the Arden gold leaf electrodes sitting on the lower lids.

● The reference electrode on the forehead.

● Signal is amplified and visualized.

Parameters

AMPLITUDE (μV)

● a-wave is measured from baseline to its trough.

● b-wave is measured from the trough of a-wave to the peak of b-wave.

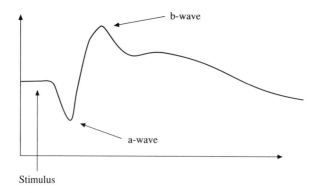

Figure 19.1 Normal standard flash ERG recording

LATENCY (MS)

- Defined as the time from the stimulus onset to the peak of the response.
- A normal flash ERG recording is shown in Figure 19.1.

Factors influencing the response

STIMULUS INTENSITY

- Increases brightness, increases the amplitude of both a- and b-waves but the latter could reach a plateau.
- The latency of peaks are reduced.
- Oscillatory potentials change positions.

FREQUENCY OF STIMULUS

- The critical flicker frequency (CFF) of rods is lower than that of cones.
- To isolate cone response, a 30 Hz flicker can be used.

COLOUR OF STIMULUS

- Red is for photopic conditions.
- Blue is for scotopic conditions.
- To isolate rod response, a weak (subcone threshold) blue light can be used in a dark-adapted eye.

ADAPTATION

- Dark adaptation increases amplitude of both a- and b-waves but also increases latency.

AGE

- Adult values reached at 2 years (smaller before then).

Clinical uses of ERG

ERG is used to:

- Confirm the diagnosis of generalized degeneration of the retina, e.g. retinitis pigmentosa.
- Assess family members of known hereditary retinal degeneration.
- Assess poor vision and nystagmus at birth.
- Assess retinal function with opaque media.
- Assess retinal function in vascular occlusion.
- Investigate unexplained poor vision.
- Monitor drug toxicity, e.g. quinine.

Common patterns of ERG in pathological conditions

RETINITIS PIGMENTOSA (RP)

- Marked reduction in amplitude of both a- and b-wave.
- Female carriers in recessive X-linked RP — 50% with abnormal ERG.

ACHROMATOPSIA (ABSENCES OF CONES)

- Normal rod ERG, but flat cones ERG.

LEBER'S CONGENITAL AMAUROSIS

- Extinguished ERG.

CONGENITAL STATIONARY NIGHT BLINDNESS

- Near normal a-wave, but absent b-wave (except AD).

DIABETIC RETINOPATHY AND CENTRAL RETINAL VEIN OCCLUSION

● Selective abolition of oscillatory potentials related to the degree of ischaemia.
● Doubtful value in assessing risks for neovascularization.

CENTRAL RETINAL ARTERY OCCLUSION

● a-wave increases in amplitude while b-wave reduces and oscillatory potentials disappear.

RETINAL DETACHMENT

● b-wave reduction proportional to area of detachment.
● Doubtful clinical prognostic value.

QUININE TOXICITY

● Reduced ERG especially to scotopic stimulation.
● ERG changes are usually permanent.

Other ERG tests

Focal ERG (FERG)

● Light directed to a small area of the retina.
● Small signal — need signal averaging machine to reduce background noise.
● Need a background light to desensitize other part of the retina.
● Clinically, only used for macular assessment.
● Might be useful in early stage of Stargardt's disease (hereditary maculopathy).

Pattern ERG (PERG)

● Use dark and light squares (checkerboard) in a TV screen.
● Can have variable size and rate of pattern reversal.
● Alternating pattern stimulates ganglion cells.
● It is more commonly used than FERG for macular assessment.
● Alternating pattern stimulates ganglion cells.

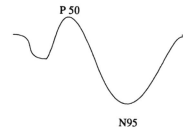

Figure 19.2 Normal pattern ERG recording

- The signals are so small that an averaging technique is required.
- It has three deflections, N35, P50 and N95.
- N indicates a negative deflection and P indicates a positive deflection.
- Only P50 and N95 have clinical values.
- N95 indicates ganglion cells function.
- P50 indicates macular function.
- Might be useful in ocular hypertension, glaucoma, optic neuritis, optic atrophy and amblyopia.
- A normal PERG recording is shown in Figure 19.2.

Electro-oculography (EOG)

- An indirect measure of the standing potential of the eye.
- Inner retina is positive as compared with the outer retina.
- The amplitude of response changes with the luminance conditions.

Standard protocol

- Electrodes are placed on either side of the eye.
- The patient moves the eyes back and forth over a specific distance.
- One electrode will become more positive than the other.
- Preadaptation period of several minutes.

- Recordings are made in the dark at 1-minute interval.
- The lowest potential (dark trough) is reached in 8–12 minutes.
- A bright light is then turned on.
- Recordings are made again at 1-minute interval.
- The highest potential (light peak) is reached in 7–10 minutes.

Parameters

- The ratio of the light peak to the dark trough (Arden index).
- The normal ratio is >180%.

Clinical uses

- In general, EOG parallels the ERG findings.
- Only exception is Best's disease (vitelliform macular dystrophy) — abnormal EOG but normal ERG.

Visual evoked cortical potentials (VECP)

- A gross electrical signal generated by the brain in response to visual stimuli.
- Commonly called visual evoked response (VER) or visual evoked potential (VEP).
- As ERG is also visual evoked response or potential, hence VECP is a better name.
- Mainly derived from the central few degrees of visual field.

Stimulus

- Flash
- Pattern (reversal or on–off) — checkerboard.

  Pattern response gives more information and is better formed.

Electrodes

- Measuring — over occipital lobe.
- Reference — ear or forehead.
- Ground — jaw or nose.

Parameters

- Latency.
- Amplitude.

Transient VECP

- Discrete negative and positive deflections.
- Most commonly used clinically.

Steady state VECP

- Elicited by increasing the temporal frequency to above 5 reversal/s or 5 Hz.
- Better in calculating latency.
- Might be useful in early glaucoma detection — debatable.

Main indications in ophthalmology

Optic nerve diseases

- Optic neuritis increase latency and decrease amplitude, often persist after resolution.

Investigation of unexplained visual loss

- Pattern VECP is usually very variable with malingering patient defocusing or refuse to fixate.

Assessment of vision in infant

- Acuity estimation using extrapolation of amplitude changes in response to check or grating size.
- Amblyopia increases latency for pattern reversal VECP.

It is important to note that Pattern VECP can be abnormal in both retinal and macular diseases. It is therefore useful to exclude these other causes before an optic nerve disease is diagnosed. A suggested test strategy for abnormal Pattern VECP is summarized in Figure 19.3.

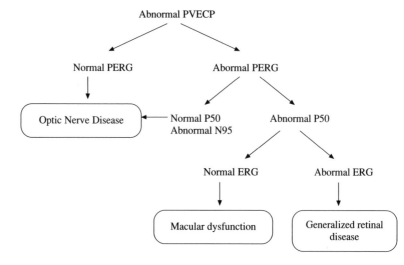

Figure 19.3 Suggested test strategy for abnormal pattern VECP (Courtesy of Dr. G. E. Holder, Moorfields Eye Hospital)

Summary of the main clinical indications of electrodiagnostic tests

EOG — Best's diseases
ERG — Generalized retinal function
PERG — Primary assessment of macular function
VECP — Optic nerve diseases

Chapter 20

Basic laser principles

Quantum theory of light

- Light has certain characteristics of a wave form.
- It can also be seen as a stream of particles.
- A particle of light energy is called a photon.
- An electron of an atom can exist at one energy level or at a higher level but at nothing in between.
- A photon can excite an electron around certain atom into the next higher energy level when it is passing through certain materials.
- It can only do that if the photon carries exactly the same energy level as the difference in energy between the two electron energy levels.

Spontaneous emission

- Energy is required to elevate the electron into the next electron energy level.
- Hence, in most material, electrons are in the lower energy level (Fig 20.1A).
- Any photon of the right level of energy can push the electron into the higher energy level (Fig 20.1B, 20.1C).
- The energized electron will fall spontaneously to its lower energy level (Fig 20.1D).
- It will then release the excess energy in the form of a photon (Fig 20.1E).
- This photon will be of exactly the same energy (i.e. same frequency, wavelength and colour) as the photon that pushed the electron to the higher level in the first place.
- This process is called spontaneous emission.
- The emitted photons go off in all directions.
- Although they are all of the same colour, they are not unidirectional nor in phase.

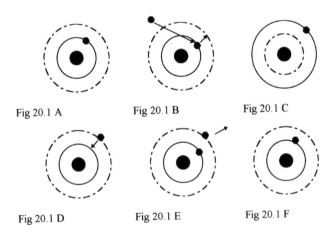

Fig 20.1 A   Fig 20.1 B   Fig 20.1 C

Fig 20.1 D   Fig 20.1 E   Fig 20.1 F

Figure 20.1 A–F Spontaneous emission

Stimulated emission

- When light of the right energy is transmitted through a medium such as the one discussed above, photons are absorbed as electrons are pushed into higher energy levels.
- The light beam is weakened by its passage through the material.
- The absorbed photons are re-emitted as the electrons fall down to the lower energy level.
- However, the re-emitted photons are released in random directions and at random times.
- The situation is different if an entering photon strikes an electron at its higher energy level (Fig 20.2A, 20.2B).
- In this case, the photon can knock the electron of its peak back to the lower energy level (Fig 20.2C, 20.2D, 20.2E).
- As the electron falls, it emits a photon.
- Thus, whereas only one photon struck the atom, two photons leave it (Fig 20.2E, 20.2F).
- That is the original photon plus the emitted photon.
- The second proton is travelling in the same direction as the first and is in phase with it.

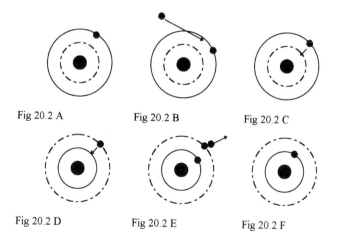

Fig 20.2 A   Fig 20.2 B   Fig 20.2 C

Fig 20.2 D   Fig 20.2 E   Fig 20.2 F

Figure 20.2 A–F Stimulated emission

- This process is called stimulated emission.
- That is the basis of laser light.
- In fact, the term laser is an acronym for Light Amplification by the Stimulated Emission of Radiation.

Thus, whether an incoming beam of light is weakened or augmented by its passage through matter depends on the proportion of atoms in that material that have their elevatable electrons in the higher energy level. If most atoms do not have many electrons in the higher level, the light beam will be weakened. If most atoms do have many electrons in the higher level, stimulated emission will occur and the light beam will be augmented as it emerges.

Population inversion

- In the natural state of matter, most electrons are at their lowest energy levels.
- One of the requirements for laser action is that the majority of elevatable electrons must be at their higher energy level before the light enters the medium.
- Such a situation is called a population inversion.
- To create a population inversion, energy must be supplied to the medium.
- In the case of solid lasers, such as the ruby or the neodymium-YAG laser, the energy may be supplied in the form of external flashes of light (by surrounding the solid crystal with a helical flash tube).
- In the case of gas lasers (such as argon, krypton and so on) the external energy may be supplied in the form of an electric current passing through the gas.
- The two possible fates of a beam of light that passes through the solid or gas of a laser.
- If a majority of the electrons are not in the higher level, the light beam will be weakened by a net loss of photons absorbed in pushing the electrons to the higher level.
- If a majority of the electrons are already at their higher level (a population inversion), the light beam will be augmented. Its photons will strike energized electrons, causing them to fall to their lower energy level.

- For each electron knocked down, a photon is released and is added to the original light beam.
- It is almost as if a chain reaction occurs, exponentially increasing the strength of the light beam.

Amplification system

- The energy of the emitted laser beam can be increased still further by causing the light beam to transverse the material multiple times.
- This is accomplished by placing a mirror over each end of the crystal or gas tube so that the distance between them is an even multiple of the laser light's wavelength.
- The light will be reflected back and forth.
- If external energy is still being supplied so that a population inversion is present, the laser beam will be amplified.
- As the photons produce by stimulated emission travel in the same direction and are in phase with the original photons that caused their emission.
- The coherent light beam continues to bounce back and forth between the two mirrors, it becomes more and more intense.
- With the two mirrors like this, no laser light will ever emerge from the apparatus.
- In the construction, one mirror must be only partially reflecting.
- The laser light can then be emerged from this end.
- Solid or gas lasers may emit continuously if the exciting energy is applied continuously.
- This output is limited in part by the heat generated in the lasing medium.
- If the exciting energy is supplied in brief pulses, laser output of higher energy level in pulses can be obtained.

Characteristics of the emitted laser beam

- It is composed of a single wavelength, in other words, monochromatic.

- All the components of the light beam are in step with one another. The laser light is said to be coherent.
- Unlike conventional light source which radiates in all directions, laser light is emitted along a single axis.
- It has high energy density.

Uses of ophthalmic lasers

Argon, krypton, dye and diode lasers

Photocoagulation

- Light energy is absorbed by ocular pigments such as melanin, haemoglobin and xanthophyll.
- This energy is converted into heat and coagulate the tissue.

The argon blue laser (488 nm) is absorbed by melanin, haemoglobin and xanthophyll. The argon green laser (515nm) has reduced absorption by xanthophyll, hence it is safer in the macular region where xanthophyll are present The krypton red laser (647 nm) is absorbed by melanin only and hence safer in the macular region, in addition, it can be used through vitreous haemorrhage. Dye laser with variable wavelengths (514–647 nm) allows the surgeon to choose the desired wavelength. The diode laser is in the infra-red range (810 nm), and allows further theoretical advantages over the krypton red laser. The diode laser is also very small and hence portable (see Table 20.1).

Table 20.1 Comparison of different thermal lasers. Percentages shown are the absorption ratios of the laser energy by various pigments.

	Argon blue	Argon green	Krypton	Diode
Wavelength (nm)	488	514	647	810
Melanin	50%	35%	20%	15%
Haemoglobin	15%	10%	3%	1%
Xanthophyll	45%	20%	5%	1%

Ophthalmic uses

- Panretinal photocoagulation for ischaemic retinae, e.g. in proliferative diabetic retinopathy or retinal vein occlusion.
- Focal photocoagulation for focal diabetic maculopathy.
- Macular grid photocoagulation for diffuse diabetic maculopathy.

- Photocoagulation of choroidal neovascularization (CNV), e.g. in age-related macular degeneration (ARMD).
- Peripheral iridotomy for closed angle glaucoma.
- Laser trabeculoplasty for open angle glaucoma.
- Cutting sutures for postoperative trabeculectomy (glaucoma surgery).
- Retinal tear repair.
- Photocoagulation in retinopathy of prematurity (ROP).

Neodymium yttrium–aluminium–garnet (Nd-YAG) laser

Photodisruption

- The laser energy is brought to a point focus.
- Any material in the minute volume at this laser's focus is ironized and a 'plasma' is formed.
- At this point, the atoms are stripped of their electrons.
- Plasma formation leads to an extremely rapid volume expansion, discharging a shock wave and significant thermal energy to the adjacent tissues.
- As it is not pigment dependent, it can be used in transparent tissues.
- The YAG laser is an infrared light at 1064 nm wavelength.

Ophthalmic uses

- Posterior capsulotomy in postoperative cataract.
- Peripheral iridotomy for closed angle glaucoma.
- Cycloablation for end stage glaucoma.
- Vitreolysis for vitreous band in proliferative diabetic retintopathy — research.
- Vitreous floaters after posterior vitreous detachment — research.

Excimer laser

Photodissociation

- Each photon has sufficient energy to break the carbon–carbon bond in organic tissues.

- The macromolecules then fall apart.
- As photons can only penetrate a few microns into the tissue, it is safe for corneal work.
- The argon/fluoride laser emits an ultraviolet wave of 193 nm.

Ophthalmic uses

- For correction of refractive error.
- Removal of superficial corneal scarring or deposits such as band keratopathy.

Index